1. It's natural to feel pain and stiffness in the joints as you get older.

2. All arthritis is the same.

3. You can get rid of arthritis by avoiding tomatoes, potatoes, and eggplant.

4. Exercise is the key to living well with arthritis.

5. You can lessen or eliminate your pain without drugs.

Answers: 1. False; 2. False; 3. False for most people; 4. True; 5. True.
Knowing the Truth About Arthritis Is the First Step in Feeling Better. And You Can Learn All the Facts, and So Much More in . . .

Living with Arthritis

Dr. Harry Shen is a physician in the Department of Rheumatic Diseases at the Hospital for Joint Disease in New York City, where he lives. He is a graduate of Cornell University and the Boston University School of Medicine. **Cheryl Solimini** is the author of four books and writes the "Pharmacy Facts" column for *Family Circle*, and the "Getting Physical" column for *New Woman*. She lives in Milford, Pennsylvania.

LIVING WITH Arthritis

*Successful Strategies to Help
Manage the Pain and Remain Active*

HARRY SHEN, M.D., AND CHERYL SOLIMINI

Illustrations by Kent Humphreys

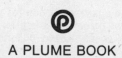

A PLUME BOOK

Thanks to Ronald Cahn for his help and advice.

PLUME
Published by the Penguin Group
Penguin Books USA Inc., 375 Hudson Street,
New York, New York 10014, U.S.A.
Penguin Books Ltd, 27 Wrights Lane, London W8 5TZ, England
Penguin Books Australia Ltd, Ringwood, Victoria, Australia
Penguin Books Canada Ltd, 10 Alcorn Avenue,
Toronto, Ontario, Canada M4V 3B2
Penguin Books (N.Z.) Ltd, 182-190 Wairau Road,
Auckland 10, New Zealand

Penguin Books Ltd, Registered Offices:
Harmondsworth, Middlesex, England

First published by Plume, an imprint of New American Library,
a division of Penguin Books USA Inc.

First Printing, August, 1993
10 9 8 7 6 5 4 3 2 1

Ⓟ REGISTERED TRADEMARK—MARCA REGISTRADA

LIBRARY OF CONGRESS CATALOGING IN PUBLICATION DATA:
Shen, Harry.
   Living with arthritis : successful strategies to help manage the
pain and remain active / Harry Shen and Cheryl Solimini.
      p. cm.
   ISBN 0-452-26997-0
   1. Arthritis—Popular works. I. Solimini, Cheryl. II. Title.
RC933.S433   1993
616.7′22—dc20   92-44844
                                                      CIP
Printed in the United States of America
Designed by Eve L. Kirch

PUBLISHER'S NOTE
The ideas, procedures, and suggestions contained in this book are not in-
tended as a substitute for consulting with your physician. All matters regarding your health require medical supervision.

Contents

CHAPTER 1

Fact vs. Fiction

Your fingers don't glide as effortlessly as they once did over the piano keys. Nothing to worry about, you think; the stiffness will probably go away. It can't be arthritis—you're only in your thirties.

You stand up from weeding in the garden, ignoring your creaky knees. Once you hit your sixties, you knew it was only a matter of time before you'd feel this way. After all, your mother had arthritis, and so did her mother. Nothing you can do about it but take a couple of aspirin to relieve the swelling.

When your doctor said that the pain in your hips was the beginning of arthritis, you were devastated. You've stayed active all your life so that you'd avoid a doddering old age, and now you'll even have to give up your daily golf game.

Everyone gets it, right? It's the first sign of old age, isn't it? You'll never again feel free from pain, will you? These are just a few of the assumptions that are made about the chronic condition known as arthritis.

Whether you've already been diagnosed with arthritis or merely suspect you have it, you probably think you know something about its symptoms and treatments. Because it's such a common disorder (one in seven Americans are affected), much of your knowledge may have come to you through word of mouth. Since arthritis has been around even longer than man or woman has walked upright, it has had plenty of time to develop its own folklore of remedies and warnings. Because these "truths" have been repeated so often, many people don't realize that much of what they've heard has been oversimplified or misstated or may not apply to their own situation.

If you haven't yet investigated the facts about arthritis on your own, you may be vulnerable to this misinformation. Arthritis is an age-old problem with no sure cure, so its sufferers are fair game for those claiming to offer a permanent solution—one that "doctors won't tell you about because they just want you to keep coming back." If you're afflicted with arthritis, it's easy to grab on to the latest "cure" if you fear you will never find relief through traditional medicine. Besides—what could it hurt?

Such thinking can be dangerous. It causes many people to forgo or delay medical care. You may avoid seeking a doctor's diagnosis, "wishing away" your aches and pains instead. Meanwhile, the disease is progressing, and the damage it causes may be irreparable. At the very least, you'll be missing out on the tried-and-true techniques and therapies that could ease your symptoms.

Here's a quick look at some of the fictions and half-truths that many people associate with arthritis. Have any of these beliefs kept you from seeking help or following through in taking control of your condition?

FICTION: It's natural to feel pain and stiffness in the joints as you get older.

FACT: There's nothing "natural" about pain and stiffness, no matter what your age. Inflammation or a loss of easy movement is a signal that something is wrong, and such symptoms should be brought to the attention of your doctor. What *is* natural is that you want to feel better, and you can. There's no reason to suffer needlessly: Arthritis is a treatable condition; in many cases, relief can be had quickly and easily. On the other hand, your aches may have nothing to do with arthritis and may be related to an even more serious ailment. You need to find out exactly what is wrong by having a medical history taken and undergoing a physical examination.

FICTION: All arthritis is the same.

FACT: There are more than 100 forms of arthritis. Some are merely uncomfortable, others crippling. They don't all respond to the same treatment. That's why an accurate diagnosis is so important. By pinpointing which type you have and how it's affecting you, your doctor can decide what therapies are right for your condition.

FICTION: Arthritis strikes only the elderly.

FACT: Don't discount arthritis as the cause of your woes just because you think you're too young. This disease isn't that selective; it can develop at any time in your life, from birth on. Some forms of arthritis surface early, then disappear in later adulthood. Nor is arthritis an inevitable consequence of aging; some older people never become arthritic.

FICTION: Arthritis is a painful, but not serious, disorder.

FACT: Because it is often viewed as simply an annoyance of old age, arthritis is rarely thought of as a major health threat. However, some forms of the disease affect not only the joints but also other parts of the body—including the skin, kidneys, heart, lungs and other vital organs. Left untreated, this damage can progress, resulting in severe disability and even death.

FICTION: Exercise will aggravate your arthritis.

FACT: Exercise can *alleviate* your arthritis, and is usually an essential part of any prescription for an arthritic patient. Strong muscles are needed to support ailing joints. In addition, specific activities can increase your mobility and reduce pain. And of course, exercise will improve your overall health.

FICTION: Living in a warm climate will cure arthritis.

FACT: Nothing "cures" arthritis. You may feel more comfortable in a balmier, drier climate—who wouldn't? But there are many considerations when planning a move, and your arthritis should be the last thing to dictate where you spend the rest of your life.

FICTION: Heat offers the best relief for your arthritis pain.

FACT: Because heat does relax muscles, a warm bath, heating pad, or hot compress will do wonders for some people, some of the time. For other people and at other times, an application of cold feels better, because it numbs the swollen area. In addition, there are many other therapies for controlling pain. After consulting with your doctor, and through trial and error, you'll discover what is best for you and when.

FICTION: You don't need a doctor's prescription. When your arthritis flares up, just take aspirin.

FACT: In arthritis treatment, aspirin is commonly used to relieve inflammation and pain; but again, it's only one of many therapies. As with any drug, aspirin has its share of side effects; it can irritate the stomach and so is not a good choice for many people. Never try to self-medicate. You should take aspirin only if your doctor recommends it.

FICTION: Arthritis means the end of your active life-style.

FACT: Tell that to dancer Cyd Charisse, who recently made her Broadway debut at age sixty-nine, or tennis great Jack Kramer, who went on to win Wimbledon after developing arthritis at age twenty-nine. Arthritis didn't stop Chopin from composing his études or Grandma Moses from starting to paint when she was in her seventies. In most cases, with proper medical attention and planning, you can continue in many of the activities you've enjoyed in the past—and even begin participating in some new ones.

FICTION: You'll get rid of your arthritis by avoiding foods that are in the nightshade family, such as tomatoes, potatoes and eggplant.

FACT: Except in the case of gout, no clear connection has been shown between a particular food or food group and any form of arthritis. Some patients swear that since giving up tomatoes or peppers their symptoms are less frequent, and there is some evidence that an allergic reaction to certain foods can trigger an arthritis flare-up. But this applies to a very small fraction of cases. A change in diet probably won't work for you, and should never be attempted without first consulting your doctor. Otherwise you may unwittingly eliminate nutrients that are important for a healthy body.

Now that you have the facts, you'll want to know more about what you can do to live—and live well—with arthritis. First you should learn as much as you can about the disease itself—what it is, what causes it and how it affects you. The next chapter provides this overview for the most common types of arthritis.

CHAPTER 2

What Is Arthritis?

When you began to notice some stiffness in your fingers, that ache in your lower back or the swelling of your knees, your first thought was probably "arthritis"—or "rheumatism," as your parents or grandparents called it. Perhaps that conjured up a picture of yourself rocking on the front porch, rubbing liniment into the sore spots and knowing when it was going to rain by the way your joints hurt. In other words, you saw yourself as helpless and old, no matter what your age.

You're not alone; many of the estimated 37 million Americans who have arthritis share your feelings. The image of this condition as an inevitable—and incurable— consequence of growing older has convinced too many of us that there is *nothing* that can be done about it. Yes, it's true that if you live long enough (knock on wood), your joints will eventually feel the strain—although arthritis can also afflict the young. What's *not* true is that you have no control over the condition.

It may be difficult for you to believe that. Your picture of arthritis probably evolved from the way this condition was viewed by previous generations. History has allowed arthritis plenty of time to develop its disheartening image. The dinosaurs had it, as evident in the remains of 200-million-year-old skeletons. Arthritis afflicted the ape-man of 2 million years ago and his descendants—Java man and Lansing man—1½ million years later. It has been found under the wrappings of Egyptian mummies dating to 8000 B.C. The public baths of the Roman Empire were built to ease the aches and pains of arthritic citizens. (The emperor at the turn of the fourth century, Diocletian, was so sympathetic to arthritis sufferers that he even excused them from paying taxes!) If you look closely at portraits from as far back as the sixteenth century, you may see the subjects' knobbed knuckles and reddened hands—an artist's rendering of arthritis. Given this disease's disreputable past, it may be easier for you to think of yourself as just another in a long line of the afflicted.

Times have changed. While arthritis has been around for millions of years, scientists have gained a true understanding of this disorder only within the past three centuries. Effective, reliable treatments have been developed just in the past fifty years. Perhaps not enough time has passed yet to improve most people's outlook on arthritis. But *you* began to change *yours* as soon as you opened this book.

Undoubtedly, the way you perceive arthritis will affect how well you can live with it. If you see it as a fate over which you have no control, it will control you: You'll limit your activities and your goals to confirm your feelings of being a victim. If you see it as just another obstacle to overcome, you will be in control: You'll chart ways to detour around discomfort without abandoning the course of your life. Numerous studies and anecdotal evidence have shown that if they take an active part in their own treatment, people with chronic and even life-threatening illnesses have the best outcome: They feel better, accomplish more, live longer. A positive attitude is not just for Pollyannas; it's vital for good health.

The first step toward action is education. When you learn all you can about arthritis, you'll find that your condition seems less mysterious and more manageable. You'll see why diagnosis and consultation with a doctor are so important, why certain treatments are better for you than others and why you need to follow those treatments exactly as directed. "Knowledge is power," wrote the philosopher Sir Francis Bacon—and you can use it to overpower arthritis.

Anatomy of a Joint

Let's start at the beginning—with the word *arthritis*. From the Greek *arthron* ("joint") and *itis* ("inflammation"), this is a very broad term that covers more than 100 of the so-called rheumatic diseases (from another Greek word, *rheuma,* or "flowing," rooted in the ancient medical belief that certain body fluids caused certain illnesses). In general, rheumatic illnesses can include inflammations of joints, muscles, ligaments or other connective tissues; some conditions are only temporary and short-term. All the arthritides are linked by pain or aching in at least one joint, and are usually chronic—lasting for a long period or recurring frequently.

Where does this discomfort come from? First, picture a healthy joint—the place where the ends of two bones meet. This could be your elbow (the rendezvous point between your upper-arm bone and the large bone of your forearm); your knee (the juncture of kneecap, thighbone, and large lower-leg bone); or any knuckle (where the short bones that make up your fingers come together). Your body has sixty-eight joints in all; most act like hinges, allowing different bones to move freely in different directions and in relation to each other.

This is possible because of the interaction of several types of tissue. *Cartilage* caps the end of each bone; the spongy yet tough material softens any impact to the joint and keeps the bones from rubbing together. The *synovium,* a membrane-lined sac that covers the joint, produces a lubricant called synovial fluid—the "grease" that keeps cartilage slippery and nourishes it as well. The *joint capsule,* a fibrous membrane, encloses the entire joint and bone ends. *Ligaments*—fibrous, rubbery bands—connect the bones of the joint and stabilize them, while still allowing them to move freely. Attached to the bones by inelastic cords called *tendons* are the *muscles,* which can contract to create the "hinge" movement of the joints. *Bursae,* small fluid-filled pouches, are strategically located at pressure points to cushion and prevent friction between these connective tissues.

What can go wrong with this well-oiled machine? Sometimes, because of an inherent defect or simple wear and tear, cartilage can become damaged, frayed or worn away completely. In other instances, the synovium may become irritated or thicken abnormally, or other tissues may be inflamed. The result, in all cases, is that the normal, smooth functioning of the joint is impaired.

One feature common to most of these conditions is inflammation. This is the body's natural reaction to injury, irritation or infection. It's responsible for the pain, redness and feeling of warmth or swelling that you notice in whatever area is touched by arthritis. It's evidence that your immune system has identified "foreign invaders" and set into motion other processes that will drive them out or destroy them. Pain is the signal from nearby nerve endings

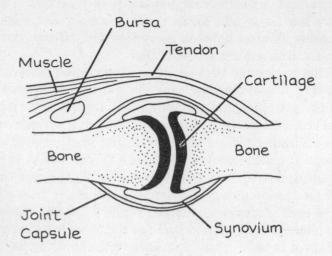

Muscle　Bursa　Tendon　Cartilage

Bone　Bone

Joint Capsule　Synovium

HEALTHY JOINT

that something is not as it should be. The redness and warmth come from the extra blood your body sends to bring nutrients, oxygen and other helpful substances to the affected tissue. In particular, one kind of leukocyte (a type of white blood cell) releases special chemicals such as *leukotrienes* and *prostaglandins,* which bring about inflammation. These substances encourage more fluids and white blood cells from surrounding tissue to rush to the affected area, where they accumulate and cause swelling.

Normally, the defenses put up by the immune system are enough to take care of the problem, and inflammation goes away after a while. In some forms of arthritis, however, whatever is affecting the tissue cannot be stopped, and the inflammation remains for a long time or returns again and again. In other cases, the inflammation process goes out of control because of a defect in the immune system itself.

When the immune system is working properly, special white blood cells called *lymphocytes* are produced to attack any unknown entity that enters the body and tries to invade healthy cells; this invader, or *antigenic material*, could be a virus, bacteria, cancer, fungus infection or any substance the body perceives as harmful. The lymphocytes come in two forms: *B cells* and *T cells*. B cells manufacture *antibodies*, the molecules that render the antigens harmless. T cells function as *helpers*, aiding the B cells or other T cells, or as suppressors to quiet down the immune system. Other T cells are cytotoxic, and can destroy infected cells.

For some people with arthritis, this defense system goes haywire. T cells may be faulty, unable to stop the creation of antibodies. The B cells may overproduce antibodies, which begin attacking healthy tissue as if the body had an allergy to itself; this condition is known as an *autoimmune disorder*. Why this happens is not clear. A particular virus may trigger an abnormal immune-system response. Certain genes may also have an influence: Human leukocyte antigens (HLAs) are genetic proteins, some of which are found on the surface of all cells, and others are on some cells of the immune system, helping to identify foreign substances. The presence or absence of specific HLAs may determine how well the immune system does its job.

In any case, people with arthritis suffer repeated cycles of inflammation. What adds insult to injury is that the tissues become even more damaged when continually bombarded with the very chemicals the body produces to help them. These substances, strong enough to destroy bacteria and other invaders, can also be destructive to normal cells over time. They can trigger abnormal changes in the tissue, eat away at cartilage and bone, weaken ligaments and tendons. Under these conditions, joints can become deformed or the bones can grow together *(fuse)*.

This is why some types of arthritis are considered "progressive": The longer the inflammation is left untreated, the more damage is done. What started out as discomforting could become disabling.

Types of Arthritis

Joint inflammation is the common link among the many forms of arthritis, but it's only a symptom, not the diagnosis, of these diseases. Some types of arthritis cause inflammation only in the joints or a particular joint. Others also involve the muscles, ligaments, tendons or other connective tissues. Some influence internal organs or the body's largest external organ—the skin. Still others are systemic, meaning that they affect nearly all parts of the body to some extent.

Before you can begin to take charge of your health, you must know about the form of arthritis you have. The most common or best-known types are described below. The scenarios that start off each section are meant to illustrate the most typical and noticeable features of the disease. Don't consider these descriptions a substitute for a proper diagnosis; *that* can only be determined through your doctor's examination.

Osteoarthritis

You feel a deep ache in one or two joints after activity, but it goes away with rest. Eventually, the pain remains even after resting and may disrupt your sleep. Cold, dampness or a change in barometric pressure aggravates it. The stiffness is most obvious when you get up in the morning or have been sitting too long.

This may be osteoarthritis (OA), the most common form of arthritis, affecting about 16 million Americans. It's often associated with aging because about 80 percent of people over fifty-five have some signs of it in their joints, but it's by no means only a disease of the elderly. Most often, those who have it never experience symptoms or disability.

The disorder, also called degenerative joint disease, originates from the gradual breakdown of joint cartilage. Why this happens is not certain. It may be due to accumulated wear and tear from everyday activity, severe or repeated injury (such as a professional athlete might sustain), a genetic defect—or a combination of these circumstances. Whatever the process, cartilage begins to split or flake off; sometimes it disappears entirely, causing the unprotected bone ends to rub together. Fragments of cartilage and bone caught in the joint space can irritate the synovium, causing inflammation. Beneath the abnormal tissue, the bone may become tough and thick, and may grow or develop lumps *(spurs)* on the outside of the joint. Though OA may make joints creaky or misshapen, the disease usually is not crippling.

The hands are a frequent site of osteoarthritis, most often in women. You may have first noticed that the joints nearest your fingernails seemed enlarged, from bony growths known as Heberden's nodes. (You may later see the same signs in the middle joints of your fingers, called Bouchard's nodes.) These knobs may not look too attractive, but they rarely interfere with your usual movements; the pain may be slight or even disappear after a while. Your grandmother or mother may have this condition too, as it seems to run in families. In fact, researchers have only recently discovered a genetic marker that may be the trigger in this and other forms of osteoarthritis. (A genetic marker is a specific gene that can be traced to a specific trait, such as eye color; unfortunately, you can also inherit certain genes that make you more susceptible to some diseases like osteoarthritis.) Generations of an Ohio family who developed OA at an early age were all found to have a faulty gene for a particular type of collagen, one of the building blocks of cartilage. So for some OA patients, these weak blocks may be responsible for the collapse in their cartilage's structure.

Osteoarthritis usually occurs in only one or two joints. Besides the hands, the neck can also be affected. Backache—the sign of OA in the lower spine—is more common in men. People who are overweight are vulnerable in the hips or knees—the weight-bearing joints. More rarely, the jaw or feet are involved. (Wrists, elbows, shoulders or ankles are less commonly touched by osteoarthritis, unless due to direct injury or some other disease.) Stress or impact on the joints seems to be the cause, but it may be that these conditions have an influence only if heredity predisposes you to OA.

Rheumatoid Arthritis

You feel more tired than usual. In the morning, it takes at least a half hour for muscle stiffness to go away, and you may even have difficulty grasping your first cup of coffee. You have pain and swelling in one or more joints that are barely noticeable at first, but gradually worsen over several days, weeks or even months. These symptoms may disappear for a while, then return. You may lose your appetite, and lose weight, or have a slight fever (not higher than 101 degrees). Eventually, movement becomes limited; joints may become deformed or "frozen" into a bent position.

Rheumatoid arthritis (RA) is a much more potentially

Osteoarthritis

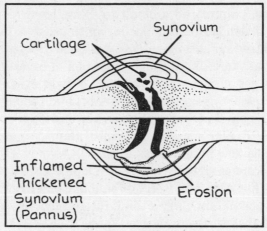

Rheumatoid Arthritis

DISEASED JOINTS

damaging disease than osteoarthritis, but not nearly as widespread. In the United States, it occurs in more than 2 million people; two to three times more women than men have RA. Most often it strikes between ages forty and sixty, but it can start at any age: Rheumatoid arthritis that begins before the age of sixteen is the most common form of chronic childhood arthritis.

The main feature of RA is *synovitis,* inflammation of the synovium, particularly where this joint membrane meets the cartilage. Constant inflammation causes changes in the synovium; it thickens and grows, as if regenerating itself to heal a wound. Inflamed synovial cells and fluid can gather to form a *pannus*—a tongue-like growth. Overgrown synovial tissue can invade the cartilage, connective tissues such as tendons, and even bone; enzymes released by the pannus destroy or weaken these joint supporting structures. Eventually, the joints can become dislocated, deformed, painful and difficult to move.

Why this inflammation occurs continues to baffle medical scientists. Emotional stress was once thought to be a cause, but more likely that is just one of several factors that can set off an arthritic episode or worsen symptoms. Recent research suggests that RA is an autoimmune disorder, triggered perhaps by an as yet undetected virus or bacteria. Genetics may come into play, as having the human leukocyte antigens HLA-DR4 and HLA-DR1 seems to increase your risk of developing rheumatoid arthritis. (For example, while only about one-fourth of the general population carries the DR4 antigen, according to some studies three-fourths of those with RA are DR4-positive. It's important to note that only a small minority of people who carry these markers becomes ill.) Other research also supports the theory that the condition may be inherited; at least one study, for instance, concluded that if one identical twin had rheumatoid arthritis, the other twin had a 50 percent chance of also developing it.

RA rarely limits itself to one area. Most often it begins in the small joints: the hands (particularly the joints at the base of the fingers), wrists, feet and knees. Later, it may affect elbows, shoulders, hips, ankles, or more rarely the neck or jaw. Joint involvement is usually symmetrical: If you have RA in one wrist, you probably have it in the other.

As the disease progresses, other body systems become affected. Lumps, called nodules, may develop under the skin at spots subject to pressure, such as at the back of the elbows or head. These are usually painless and often disappear, but can sometimes become sore or infected. Inflammation may spread to connective tissues far beyond the joints. Damage can also occur to the spleen or other organs. Nerves may be pinched by swollen tissue, as happens in carpal tunnel syndrome, a disorder marked by pain in the wrist and numbness in the fingers. Chest pains or breathing difficulties can mean that the heart or lungs are involved—complications that can be fatal.

Fortunately, with early and effective treatment most cases of rheumatoid arthritis will not progress that far. Less than 10 percent of RA patients become completely disabled—confined to bed or a wheelchair for life. More often symptoms, mild or severe, will come and go: Remissions can last for weeks, months or even years; these are followed by *flares* (or flare-ups), periods when pain and discomfort reappear or worsen.

Gout

In your sleep or upon rising in the morning, sudden, intense pain stabs at your big toe. The joint is hot, red and swollen for a few hours or days or maybe weeks, but eventually all symptoms subside . . . until the next attack months or years later.

Many people think of gout as an illness out of history—not one that today affects about 2 million Americans, 80 percent of them male. It's the third most common form of arthritis, but the easiest to detect and treat. In men, the disorder begins during the thirties or forties; nearly all women with gout develop it after menopause.

Gout has been called the "disease of kings," associated with an overindulgence in rich food and wine. However, many of the people who suffer from it can hardly afford a kingly diet. The real problem is a defect in the body's ability to process uric acid. This acid is a normal by-product of the digestion of purines (a compound found in proteins); it circulates through the bloodstream, is filtered out by the kidneys and is then passed in the urine. However, some people produce too much acid and cannot get rid of it fast enough; in some cases, the kidneys are unable to remove it efficiently. (Gout can also result from other conditions that directly prevent the kidneys from functioning properly, including lead poisoning, overuse of diuretics or diseases such as severe diabetes.) A defect in the body's chemistry—an enzyme mutation—allows uric acid to build up in the blood; it eventually forms urate crystals, which enter and irritate the synovium of some joints. Not everyone who has high blood levels of uric acid will get gout. The condition seems to be hereditary; if someone in your family has had it, you have about a 40 percent chance of developing it.

For reasons not yet understood, gout targets only a few specific joints—most often the bunion joint of the big toe, and sometimes other foot joints, the ankles, knees, elbows, wrists and fingers, but rarely the shoulders, hips or lower spine. If gout is not treated, urate crystals can collect into masses called *tophi*, which deposit in cartilage, synovium, tendons, soft tissue or anywhere else on the body. These appear as bulbous lumps on ears, fingers, hands, knees, feet or near the elbows or Achilles tendons. Kidneys can also be damaged trying to handle the excess uric acid. Except in the advanced stage of gout, symptoms flare, then abate for a time. Attacks may be provoked by stress, surgery, infections, overeating, alcohol or certain drugs like diuretics (often used to treat high blood pressure).

Ankylosing Spondylitis

You wake up with low back pain or stiffness that fades as you become more active throughout the day. This discomfort persists for more than three months and may disrupt your sleep. Lying down or sitting for more than two hours worsens symptoms. When you inhale, you may feel a pain in your chest. You also may feel tired and be losing weight.

From the Greek *ankylos* ("crooked") and *spondylos* ("vertebra"), ankylosing spondylitis, or AS, can easily be confused with mechanical back pain—the nonarthritic condition that usually results from unaccustomed strain on the spine, such as when hoisting a heavy object or playing a sport. (The table that follows can help you tell the difference between simple backache and AS.) Because of this "mistaken identity" in the past, AS is believed to be more common than previously thought. In the United States, it afflicts about 1 in 1,000 before age forty. Men make up 80 to 90 percent of these AS cases, but that estimate may be misleading: Women often have much milder symptoms, which may never be diagnosed as AS. Children, mostly boys, account for one in twenty cases.

In AS, inflammation settles at the points where a ligament, tendon or joint capsule attaches to joint bones, usually in the spine. Rather than weakening or eroding, the joint produces more bone, which grows to bridge the gap between the small bones of the back, or vertebrae. Once the bone ends grow together, or *fuse*, the joint becomes immovable.

As with most of the arthritic diseases, the cause of AS is unclear. Like Reiter's syndrome and psoriatic arthritis (two similar inflammations of the spinal joints, described in "Other Arthritic Conditions" later in this chapter), AS has a strong link to the genetic marker HLA-B27. However, only 20 percent of people with B27 will actually develop AS. Your odds increase if another member of your family has the disease. Still, this inherited tendency must be activated in some way; scientists are still searching for the switch.

Ankylosing spondylitis begins with pain in the lower

back, spreading upward to the middle and upper back and neck, and sometimes down into the buttocks or thighs. For about 20 percent of AS sufferers, the first arthritic symptoms occur in the hips, shoulders or other joints. As AS progresses, these joints as well as the spine are affected. Inflammation often strikes tendons in the chest (which causes the breathing pain) and heels. In later stages of AS, the eyes and prostate gland can become inflamed; heart and lungs can also be affected. With early treatment, these complications and total fusion of the spine can be headed off.

Comparison of Simple Back Pain and AS

	Mechanical Back Pain	Ankylosing Spondylitis
Onset	Sudden	Gradual
Age	15–90	Under 40
History	Occasional symptoms, linked to past injury or strain	Persistent (more than 3 months), with no past injury
Family history	No	Yes
Location of pain	Lower back	Lower to upper back, buttocks
Morning stiffness	Mild	Prolonged
Effect of exercise	Worsens pain	Relieves pain
Effect of rest	Relieves pain	Worsens pain
Disturbs sleep	Rarely	Frequently

Systemic Lupus Erythematosus

Two or more of your smaller joints become tender, swollen and red. A butterfly-shaped rash spreads over the bridge of your nose and cheeks, and other rashes may surface on skin exposed to sunlight. You feel very tired, even exhausted, with a fever of 101 or higher and muscle ache. Deep breathing or coughing may bring on a sharp pain in your chest. You seem to have lost some weight recently for no apparent reason, and you notice you're also losing your hair—too many strands are falling out when you comb or wash it.

Systemic lupus erythematosus (also known as SLE or lupus) afflicts nine times as many women as men, and usually starts in the childbearing years—between ages fifteen and thirty-five. Though it is a rare condition (about 1 in 2,000 have it), incidence seems to be increasing—probably because tests developed only in the past few decades have made it easier for doctors to detect lupus. More importantly, what was once a usually fatal disease can now be controlled by new treatments available.

In lupus, connective tissues throughout the body become inflamed. What causes this inflammation is unknown, but medical scientists believe that several factors may work together. Stress, sunlight or hormone production may have an influence; some drugs, such as the high blood pressure medication hydralazine and the heart drug procainamide, can create a lupus-like disease in certain people. Lupus also tends to run in families, and the presence of the genetic markers HLA-DR2 and DR3 points to a higher risk of developing it. Some patients with lupus also lack a particular protein usually found in blood enzymes that are involved in the immune response.

Lupus is almost surely an autoimmune disorder: Researchers have found that those with SLE produce antinuclear antibodies, which mistakenly attach themselves to substances in the nuclei of cells, such as DNA (the molecules that contain genetic information). (Anti-DNA antigens can deposit in kidneys and cause kidney disease in lupus patients.) As in rheumatoid arthritis, an unknown virus may trigger this immune-system defect, but only for those already genetically susceptible to lupus.

Sometimes just the skin is affected—a less damaging condition known as *discoid lupus*. But as its name indicates, true SLE is systemic—meaning that it involves the entire body. Sores can form on the inside of the mouth and nose. Arthritic pain commonly develops in the knuckles and middle joints of the fingers, the knees and the wrists, and less often in the ankles, elbows and shoulders. Usually, these joints are not deformed by the disease. In later stages of lupus, inflammation reaches the linings of the heart and lungs; the kidneys and nervous system could also become damaged. Fortunately, most cases of lupus are mild. Even in severe cases, early detection and treatment can prevent the disease from spreading to organs and other vital systems.

Scleroderma

When you wake up in the morning, your face, hands or feet feel puffy, and tingly or numb, with the skin taut and shiny. When you're cold or under emotional stress, your fingers hurt and look "frostbitten," the color changing to blue, then deathly pale. You may feel weak and have pain or stiffness in a few joints. After a few weeks or months, the skin on your fingers, hands, face and arms becomes thick and hard.

Scleroderma (literally "hard skin") is an uncommon rheumatic disease, but can be life-threatening. It occurs in an estimated three to twelve persons in every million. Two

to three times more women than men have it. While scleroderma can strike at any age, more often it begins between
thirty and sixty. The condition is rare among children and
within families.

Connective tissue is the chief target of scleroderma.
First, the tiny blood vessels of the body become inflamed.
What happens next is still uncertain; most experts believe
that the body begins overproducing collagen, the fibrous
protein which is usually found in connective tissue but
which is also a component of scar tissue. This collagen
deposits in the skin and other areas, where it thickens and
hardens.

Scleroderma is considered an autoimmune disorder:
Something triggers the B cells to produce antibodies and
also to stimulate the production of collagen. The activating agent is unknown, but may be a chemical or environ-
mental factor. For instance, workers exposed to vinyl
chloride (a gas used in the making of some plastics), people
who take bleomycin (a cancer drug) or L-tryptophan (an
amino acid supplement wrongly promoted to cure sleeping
difficulties), and miners who breathe in silica dust have
been known to come down with a scleroderma-like condition. This syndrome has also been noted in a few cases
involving silicone breast implants.

Unlike most arthritic diseases, scleroderma does not
often damage the joints directly; some joints—usually the
hands—may feel stiff or creaky because of thickening
skin. In some severe cases, muscles may contract
permanently—"freezing" a joint into a bent position, to
crippling effect. The frostbite-like symptoms in fingers
—called *Raynaud's phenomenon*—are much more common and usually the first sign of scleroderma. These
symptoms can occur in otherwise healthy people. However, the more serious concern lies in the scarring of organ

tissues. If the disease progresses, the esophagus, intestinal tract, kidneys, heart and lungs can be affected and these systems may fail—with deadly consequences.

Fortunately, scleroderma is mild in most people. Though skin will remain thickened for three to fifteen years, eventually it softens a bit and may even return to almost normal.

Juvenile Arthritis

Your child's temperature may swing from normal to as high as 103 throughout the day. She doesn't show as much interest in food, and may be losing weight. For several weeks, her knee has been swollen, but she may not complain that it hurts. A blotchy, red rash may appear over her body, arms and legs in the morning, only to subside later in the day. One or both of her eyes may be red too, and painful. When you check her neck and underarms, you feel swelling in the lymph glands.

Juvenile arthritis is a catchall term for the many different forms of arthritis—most often rheumatoid, ankylosing spondylitis and lupus—that can afflict youngsters before age sixteen. These diseases rarely occur before age six months; some types have peak periods of onset—between ages one and three, or from eight to twelve. It has been estimated that up to 250,000 children in the United States have arthritis. Two to three times more girls have rheumatoid arthritis; boys are more likely to have AS.

When any of these arthritic conditions develops in a child, it begins and progresses differently than it does in an adult. For instance, a child with AS may have pain in the buttocks or legs first rather than the lower back. The symptoms in the first paragraph describe the most common of the chronic childhood illnesses, *juvenile rheumatoid arthritis* (JRA). The systemic form of JRA—which can involve the heart, lungs and blood—is known as *Still's disease*, and only affects children.

In JRA, only one joint or as many as four or more may be involved—in particular, the knees, ankles, elbows and neck. Fortunately, damage is not often permanent. However, other consequences are more serious: Some types of JRA can cause eye inflammation that ends in blindness; slowed growth can prevent a child from reaching her potential height and can cause deformity of the jaw or limbs.

About 70 to 90 percent of children who have JRA recover with little or no disability. Complete remission is possible, most usually if the illness has lasted less than seven years. For most children who have had JRA, arthritis will not resurface in adulthood. Proper diagnosis and treatment are vital to the psychological as well as physical health of a child with an arthritic condition.

Other Arthritic Conditions

Psoriatic arthritis affects about 5 percent of those who have psoriasis. Similar to that dermatological disorder, this condition causes scaly red patches to form on different areas of the skin, especially on knees and elbows and near fingernails. A finger or toe may become completely swollen—the so-called "sausage digit." Like ankylosing spondylitis, psoriatic arthritis can be accompanied by back pain and is an inherited disease linked to HLA-B27 and other HLA markers.

Reiter's syndrome is another of the spondyloarthropathies—diseases of the spinal joints. Other symptoms include skin rash; arthritis in the feet, knees or ankles; and inflammations of the eye and urethra (the duct that drains urine from the bladder). Men—the disease's most frequent victims—may notice a watery or pus-like discharge from the penis. Reiter's is triggered by certain bacteria, which can be acquired through sexual contact or as a result of dysentery (severe diarrhea caused by unfriendly organisms in the bowels). However, the disease strikes those with a genetic susceptibility—usually HLA-B27 and related markers. Some people with acquired immune deficiency syndrome (AIDS) develop a Reiter's-type arthritis.

A virus, bacteria or fungus is at the root of *infectious arthritis*. Most vulnerable are people whose immune systems have already been weakened by another condition such as diabetes, sickle-cell anemia, kidney disease, alcoholism or other forms of arthritis, or by medications such as those used in cancer therapy. Infectious arthritis will usually start with fever, chills and inflammation of just one or a few joints, usually a knee, hip, ankle or shoulder, though any joint is at risk. Depending on the cause, joint damage can be rapid. However, unlike most arthritic disorders, the infectious type can be cured if the infecting agent is identified and treated as soon as possible.

Most people are unaware that *Lyme disease* is also a form of infectious arthritis. It starts with the bite of a bacteria-infected deer tick, as tiny as the head of a pin. In three to thirty days, its victim may develop a bull's-eye rash (the pale, raised bite site surrounded by reddened skin) and flu-like symptoms: headache, fever, aching muscles and joints, swollen glands. Later, arthritis may appear in the knees, hips, shoulders and some other joints; the heart and nervous system can also be affected. In its early stages the disease can mimic other disorders; even the telltale rash shows up in only about 60 percent of victims. On the other hand, some people who test positive for Lyme disease actually may have lupus or another autoimmune disorder. Fortunately, if Lyme disease is caught early, it can be easily cleared up with antibiotics. Scientists recently determined that chronic Lyme arthritis, which affects only a small minority of patients, may be an inherited susceptibility, traced to the genetic marker HLA-DR4 or HLA-DR2. This genetic connection may explain why only 10 percent of those with untreated Lyme disease develop this condition.

Like gout, *pseudogout* is caused by the deposit of crystals in the joints—in this case, calcium pyrophosphate dihydrate crystals. Unlike gout, the most frequent site of attack is the knee, which becomes hot, red and stiff; the wrist, ankle, elbow, shoulder and hip are other areas of inflammation. Pseudogout also appears later than gout, often after age seventy.

In *Sjögren's syndrome*, the glands that produce tears and saliva become inflamed, leaving the eyes and mouth dry. Eyes may be red, itchy or painful; vision may cloud and sores may form on the corneas. Swallowing or chewing may be difficult; the tongue and corners of the mouth may develop cracks or sores, and teeth may be riddled with cavities. Patients usually have a mild arthritis. While this autoimmune disorder can occur by itself, often it is also found in those with rheumatoid arthritis, scleroderma or lupus. Recent reports suggest that women with silicone implants may develop a Sjögren's-like illness.

Pain while chewing, general aches and pains, throbbing headaches, tenderness in the neck, head or temple, and sudden or occasional vision loss may be signs of *temporal arteritis*. This condition results from inflammation of certain arteries that supply blood to the upper body. It usually strikes after age fifty and often after seventy.

Rather than affecting the joint itself, *bursitis* and *tendonitis*, as their names imply, are inflammations of the bursa and tendon, respectively. They often occur after repeated or sudden stress on a joint—when playing a sport, for instance, or lifting a heavy weight. These common ailments, which include "housemaid's knee" and "tennis elbow," usually are not chronic and rarely cause permanent damage. However, recurring tendonitis can also be a sign of ankylosing spondylitis.

As you can see, the many causes and symptoms of arthritis make it impossible to offer a one-size-fits-all approach to treatment. Often even the same form of the disease behaves differently in different people. In the earliest stages, some types are very similar to others, or can be mistaken for other nonarthritic conditions. How do you know precisely which arthritis is affecting you? The next chapter explains how your doctor will make the diagnosis.

CHAPTER 3

Making the Diagnosis

Perhaps now that you know more about the many rheumatic diseases and their effects, you're sure you have arthritis . . . or you're sure you don't. Maybe your symptoms don't precisely match those for any of the disorders, or you have symptoms that weren't described. Maybe you don't feel *that* bad, or you still think your problems will just go away in time. Whatever your conclusions, you should not ignore the discomfort that led you to consult this book. Only a physician can confirm or rule out the possibility of arthritis or any other illness; only a doctor can guide you in treatment.

Seeking medical help is often the most difficult step for many people, no matter how much they're suffering. You may lack transportation to the doctor's office or have few health-care options close to your hometown. You may be concerned about the expense, particularly if you don't have medical insurance. You may be frightened at the thought of hearing bad news, putting off your appointment as long as possible. Or it may be that you just don't trust doctors—never have. These reasons keep too many people from receiving treatment until the pain cannot be ignored or they are hospitalized.

What you don't know *can* hurt you. You must make your health a priority, or the cost—physical, financial and psychological—could be immeasurable.

It has been estimated that patients currently under treatment for arthritis waited, on average, *four years* from the onset of symptoms before seeking a physician's advice. In that time, extensive, irreparable damage can be done. As you learned in Chapter 2, constant or recurring inflammation has a cumulative effect on joints as well as organs and other tissues affected by arthritis. The longer the inflammation is out of control, the further the disease can progress.

In order to interrupt the cycle of inflammation and prevent additional harm, your doctor must prescribe treatment appropriate to your condition. As pointed out previously, proper treatment depends on the form of arthritis you have. And that depends on an accurate diagnosis, arrived at by your physician using evidence from your medical history, a physical examination and certain diagnostic tests.

Early Warning Signs

The sooner you bring your complaints to your doctor's attention, the better your chances of stopping the disease in its tracks. How do you know whether your complaints deserve serious consideration? Some of the more obvious symptoms that were outlined in the preceding chapter may not surface until the disease has already taken hold. Don't wait until then—be alert to these early warning signs:

1. You have swelling in one or more joints. You may have only slight puffiness, or may notice that a ring, your wristwatch or shoes, for instance, feel tighter than before.
2. Your joints or muscles feel stiff, and the stiffness lasts for more than an hour.
3. A joint feels painful or sensitive to touch.
4. You're unable to move a joint normally. For instance, you can no longer raise your arm above your head, or cannot completely straighten your elbow or knee.
5. The joint looks red or feels warm or hot.
6. Your joint pain is accompanied by fever or a feeling of weakness, or by weight loss not connected to an attempt to diet.

If you've experienced any of these symptoms for more than two weeks, it's time to see your doctor.

In the Doctor's Office

Your regular family physician can usually perform the evaluations needed to diagnose arthritis. However, if your doctor is uncertain of the diagnosis or does not have access to or experience with certain tests, or if your symptoms are severe or the disease continues to progress, your doctor may refer you to another physician—probably a rheumatologist, a specialist in rheumatic diseases. Remember, too, that *you* should feel confident that you're receiving appropriate care. If you're dissatisfied with your doctor's treatment—perhaps you think he or she is not sufficiently qualified, or your symptoms have been dismissed as "old age"—you may ask to be referred to a specialist. You can also locate one yourself through your local medical board or chapter of the Arthritis Foundation (also see "General Resources" in Chapter 12).

Before any doctor examines you, he or she will ask about your symptoms and other medical history. These questions will enable the doctor to decide how to begin your physical examination and which tests to administer. It may help you both if you make note of what has been bothering you *before* you enter the doctor's office: Anxiety over the visit or concern that you're taking up too much of the doctor's time can influence how well you convey this important information to your physician. Also, because arthritis pain often comes and goes, chances are that by the time of your appointment, you may not be feeling so poorly and may minimize your concern. Writing down symptoms when you're aware of them will help ensure that you don't forget any details. To help you prepare, here are some areas that may be covered in your doctor's questioning:

- When did you first notice symptoms? Did they go away, only to return after a time, or are you in discomfort every day?
- Was pain sudden, or did it seem to come on gradually, over several days or weeks or longer?
- Did your symptoms occur around the same time as an injury, illness or emotional upset (such as a death in your family, job loss, a move to a new home)?
- Where do you feel pain? Is it in more than one joint? Does it seem to travel from joint to joint or radiate to other parts of your body, rather than ache in one area each time? Is it in one or both sides of your body—for instance, in one or both wrists?
- Is the pain sharp or dull, burning or throbbing? How long does it last?

- At what point of the day are symptoms most notice-able—upon rising, in the evening, during the night? Does it seem to take you longer to get going in the morning?
- What conditions aggravate your symptoms? Are you bothered by heat or cold, inclement weather, inactivity or exercise?
- Are you feeling unusually weak or tired even though you're getting plenty of rest and are not under stress? Are your symptoms affecting your appetite? Are they disturbing your sleep?
- Besides joint pain, have you had other health problems: skin rash, difficulty breathing or chest pains, diarrhea or constipation?
- Are there activities you can't do now that you had little trouble with before symptoms began, such as standing or sitting for long periods, walking, buttoning or putting on your coat, brushing your hair?
- Has anyone else in your family ever had similar symptoms? (If you're not sure, other relatives may be able to help you fill in missing family medical history.)
- Are you currently taking any drugs? (Medications often create certain symptoms or mask others, which can interfere with an accurate diagnosis. Be sure to mention not only prescription medicines but also nonprescription products such as antacids, cold remedies or aspirin. You should also be prepared to discuss your use of alcoholic beverages and illegal substances such as marijuana and cocaine.)

After questioning and a general physical examination, your physician will direct his or her attention to your joints, gently pressing on them to detect swelling, tenderness or deformity. You may then be asked to walk across the room or perform certain movements so that the doctor can see whether joint motion is limited or painful. In addition, the doctor may manipulate the joints, taking them as far as possible through their *range of motion*—the full extent that any joint can move normally at different angles and directions. Depending on which form of arthritis he or she suspects, your doctor may also test your muscle strength and tendon reflexes.

Diagnostic Testing

Often a medical history and physical are all that's necessary for your physician to come up with a diagnosis. In other cases, you may need to visit your doctor on several occasions so that he or she can chart a pattern of your condition. To confirm the diagnosis or to differentiate among some forms of arthritis, your physician is likely to order one or a few diagnostic tests, the most common of which follow. These tests alone cannot be performed to render a diagnosis, but must be evaluated in relation to your reported symptoms.

Blood Tests

A sample of blood may be pricked from your fingertip or, more likely, taken by syringe from a vein on the inside of one elbow. The components of the blood can then be examined to reveal a number of different characteristics.

Usually the first test is a *complete blood count*, or CBC. This simple screening procedure is used to measure the number of oxygen-carrying red blood cells (erythrocytes) as well as the level of hemoglobin (the chemical found in red blood cells that actually transports the oxygen to all cells), and the amount of disease-fighting white blood cells (leukocytes and lymphocytes). Sometimes the platelets, the blood cells responsible for clotting, will also be counted. A low level of hemoglobin or red blood cells indicates a type of anemia that results from chronic inflammation, found in certain types of arthritis such as RA, lupus, ankylosing spondylitis, psoriatic arthritis and Reiter's syndrome, but not in osteoarthritis. An above-normal number of white blood cells may point to an infection, such as infectious arthritis, and can also occur in gout and other forms of inflammatory arthritis. A low white cell count is common in lupus. The CBC may be used in later visits to check on your progress and also to monitor side effects of drug therapy, as some medications used in arthritis treatment can also lower white cell or platelet levels.

Inflammation can also be measured by *erythrocyte sedimentation rate*, also known as ESR or sed rate. Blood is collected in a long glass tube and left to settle for an hour. At the end of that time, the technician notes the volume of red blood cells that have separated from surrounding plasma—the clear, nutrient-rich blood fluid in which the red cells are normally suspended—and fallen to the bottom of the tube. The higher the ESR, the greater the degree of inflammation. While this does not indicate arthritis specifically, it can help to distinguish between rheumatoid arthritis (high ESR) and osteoarthritis (low ESR). During treatment, a change in ESR can be used to chart the course of your condition. However, a rise in ESR can also be caused by relatively minor problems, such as a cold or pregnancy.

Blood can also be tested for abnormal antibodies that are often present in some arthritic conditions. One such antibody is the *rheumatoid factor* (RF), which attaches to another antibody, gamma globulin. RF is found in 90 percent of patients with Sjögren's syndrome, in 80 percent of those with rheumatoid arthritis, in 30 percent of lupus patients, and in some cases of scleroderma. However, it is also seen in those with severe chronic infections, such as chronic tuberculosis. Antinuclear antibody (ANA) tests can detect the presence of the antibody that binds to certain substances in the nuclei of cells. Specific ANAs point to different forms of arthritis—such as the anti-DNA ANAs common in lupus. ANAs are found in 95 percent of people with lupus, in up to 80 percent of those with scleroderma, and in up to 80 percent of people who have Sjögren's syndrome. ANAs have also been seen in some cases of rheumatoid arthritis. On the other hand, 5 percent of people over age sixty-five have ANAs without having any autoimmune disease. ANA testing is usually performed as a screening procedure.

A *complement test* measures the amount of certain blood enzymes, called complement proteins, that are involved in the immune-system response. Levels of these enzymes are more likely to be low if you have active lupus (particularly if the disease has already begun affecting your kidneys), Sjögren's syndrome or one of a few other arthritic conditions. The test may be repeated periodically to chart the course of the disease.

When muscles are damaged, they release some of their enzymes into the bloodstream. A *muscle enzyme test* may be given when your doctor suspects polymyositis, a rheumatic disease marked by weakness of the shoulder or hip muscles, and arthritis in small joints; this condition can sometimes accompany lupus, rheumatoid arthritis or scleroderma. The presence of these enzymes in the blood can also indicate dermatomyositis, a similar disorder that in addition causes red patches to form on the face or over knuckles, knees or elbows. However, enzyme levels can also be high if you have heart disease, take certain drugs or perform heavy manual labor.

A *creatinine test* measures the blood level of creatinine, a compound released as a waste product by the muscles. But rather than indicating muscle damage, high levels of creatinine point to malfunctioning kidneys, which may not be filtering and excreting creatinine efficiently.

To confirm a diagnosis of gout, a *uric acid test* can be performed on a blood sample. However, if you're taking a diuretic (water pill) for high blood pressure or weight loss, you can also have higher than normal uric acid levels.

X Rays

Your doctor may order X rays of a few joints to aid the diagnosis or to determine the severity of damage. To get these negative-image pictures of your bones, you'll be exposed to short bursts of radiation aimed at a limited area. These radiographs can reveal the bony spurs of osteoarthritis, the spinal changes in ankylosing spondylitis or the calcium crystals that identify pseudogout, among other conditions. Often, though, in early stages of disease, damage is not extensive enough to be seen on the X ray; or a joint can appear abnormal yet create no symptoms. X rays, then, may be more useful for checking on the progress of disease.

Other methods of joint "imaging" can provide sharper detail when needed. In *arthrography*, a dye or air is injected in the joint space before an X ray; it gives the physician a clearer picture of damaged cartilage and synovial lining. Both *magnetic resonance imaging* (MRI) and *computed tomography* (CT) take cross-sectional views of the joint area; each has its use in detecting certain problems, such as tearing of tendons and ligaments, or changes in the synovium and spinal disks. Like X rays, CT uses radiation, which can increase your cancer risk if you must undergo repeated exposures. MRI uses high-power magnets in the imaging process, so it's not suitable for patients with pacemakers; the MRI scan, during which you must lie still for a time in a large, close-fitting cylinder, may be disturbing if you're claustrophobic. *Myelography*—a technique for X-raying the spine—may be used before surgery to more precisely pinpoint some problems, but it's rapidly being replaced by CT scanning, which is proving just as reliable for most cases. In some circumstances, a doctor may order *both* CT and a myelogram.

Joint Aspiration

In this examination, synovial fluid is drawn into a syringe through a needle inserted into the joint space. Aspiration is often the quickest and simplest way to diagnose many arthritic disorders. The fluid can be studied to determine such factors as white blood cell count, the presence or absence of bacteria or other infection, and the presence of crystals (pseudogout or gout) or cartilage fragments (osteoarthritis). The density, color or clarity of the fluid can also give clues to certain diseases.

Urinalysis

This test checks for red blood cells or protein in the urine—an indication of kidney damage that can occur in some diseases like lupus and scleroderma. A urine sample may be taken on your first office visit, and then at later intervals to monitor the disease's progress or the effect of

certain arthritis drugs, such as gold salts and penicillamine, which are also known to affect kidney functioning.

Biopsy

Samples of different tissues can be subjected to several
tests that can help in diagnosing or monitoring a rheumatic disease. In this procedure, a small amount of tissue
is removed either by surgical incision, scraping with a
scalpel or extracting with a special needle; it is then examined under a microscope. Skin samples, for example, can be
helpful in finding systemic diseases such as lupus, scleroderma, or psoriatic arthritis. Muscle fibers may be studied
when polymyositis is suspected. Depending on the disease,
tissue may be taken from synovial membranes, lymph
nodes or blood vessels. Kidney biopsy is often performed
on lupus patients. Liver or lung biopsies are done rarely,
because of the risk of complications. Some biopsies can be
done in the doctor's office; others may require a hospital
stay.

Arthroscopy

When a medical history, X ray and other laboratory
procedures do not lead to a clear diagnosis, your doctor
may decide to view your joint from the inside, through a
periscope-like device inserted into the joint space. This
procedure usually takes place in a hospital operating
room, while you are under general or local anesthesia.
Through the arthroscope, the doctor can also take a photograph for later examination, remove a tissue sample for
biopsy or even perform surgery using specialized equipment (see Chapter 8, "Opting for Surgery").

Electromyogram (EMG)

This test measures the electrical impulses from your muscles (similar to the way an electrocardiogram reads the electrical patterns of your heart), and is usually paired with a nerve conduction study, a test of electrical impulses of the nerves. In rheumatic diseases that involve the muscles, such as polymyositis and dermatomyositis, changes in the EMG can measure the extent of damage. In some cases of inflammatory arthritis, nerves may have been directly damaged; in other conditions, such as those that involve spinal disks, nerves may be compressed by the affected joints.

Ultrasound

This technique uses high-frequency sound waves to develop an image of certain soft tissues. Though not yet in wide use for evaluating arthritic conditions, ultrasound can spot thickened synovium, roughened cartilage and damage to organs that can result from some forms of arthritis.

Tissue Typing

Cells can also be examined for the presence of certain human leukocyte antigens—such as HLA-B27 in ankylosing spondylitis. As yet, these tests are too time-consuming and expensive for routine evaluation and are used only in research.

As indicated in the descriptions above, some tests may be administered only on your first visit, or in subsequent visits as your doctor refines his or her diagnosis. Others may be used at later stages of the disease to spot the extent of damage to tissues. Depending on the arthritis and its treatment, some tests may be given every few months, to keep an eye on the disease's progress or to be sure that the side effects of medications are not creating other health problems. When very strong drugs are prescribed (see Chapter 7, "Using Medications"), you may be subject to certain tests every month, or blood and urine samples may be taken each week.

Once your doctor is satisfied with the diagnosis, you can work together to outline a treatment program that fits into your life. How well you comply with your doctor's guidelines depends a great deal on how well you can communicate your new needs and concerns to your "support network": family, friends, your employer and colleagues, as well as your physician. Your condition may affect you, and them, in ways you never anticipated. The next chapter discusses some of these areas and offers strategies for coping.

CHAPTER 4

How Arthritis Affects You and Your Family

The impact that a diagnosis of arthritis will have on you depends on the type and severity of your condition. If your symptoms are mild, they may interfere little with your day-to-day activities. But you still may discover that having a chronic illness changes the focus of your life. Where before your work may have occupied much of your time and thoughts, now you must make your health a priority to ensure that your arthritis does not worsen. You may have to follow a medication or physical therapy schedule, and you will have to consider how to fit these new regimens into your old lifestyle.

What may be less apparent is the impact the disease has on you psychologically. Many people's first reaction upon learning of a chronic illness is shock: *How can this happen to me?* You may feel powerless or you may feel nothing— emotionally paralyzed. Once this phase passes, you may avoid thinking about your problem entirely, or may even deny that you have one. (At this point, many people often consult one doctor after another, hoping to be told that nothing is wrong or that there is a quick cure.) As symptoms force you to deal with what's happening to you, depression may set in: You may feel sad, listless (mentally and physically), unable to enjoy what used to give you pleasure. You may also experience anxiety—a nameless fear or an uneasiness that you can't seem to put a finger on. Anger may be another of your reactions: *Why me?* Your emotions may run in cycles, leading you back to depression.

You must recognize that your feelings are natural—and that they may return again and again during the course of your illness as new problems or obstacles surface. Eventually, though, you'll come around to the stage of accommodation and adjustment. You'll accept that you have arthritis and direct your energy toward dealing with the situation. You know you must work with your doctor and follow through with your therapies if you want to have control over your condition.

But even after you've come to terms with your medical needs, the realities of living with a chronic illness can still take their toll on other areas of your life: your personal relationships, job performance, finances. Because family, friends and colleagues can't *see* your pain, they might not be able to understand why you may have to limit your activities. Even loved ones may misinterpret your moods—which can shift according to the ebb and flow of your arthritis—as a reflection of your feelings for them. The cost of treatment can strain more than your bank account, if your family is forced to make sacrifices to help meet the expenses of your illness. However, if you anticipate these problems, you can overcome them too—and you don't have to do it alone.

Many medical centers that treat arthritis can offer a "team" approach. Whatever your concerns, your primary physician should be able to refer you to someone who can help—for instance, a physiatrist (a doctor trained in physical rehabilitation), physical therapist, occupational therapist, psychologist, pain management specialist, social worker or sexual counselor. (Health-care organizations, in particular your local chapter of the Arthritis Foundation, can also aid you in locating appropriate services.) These professionals can give you practical guidance in resolving difficulties you or others may be facing because of your illness. That's why it's so important that you alert your doctor to any problem arising from your arthritis, even if it doesn't seem directly related to the doctor's field of expertise.

Of course, you must be willing to discuss topics that might make you uncomfortable. You can prepare for a talk with your physician by thinking through, and even writing down, the problems you're experiencing. To get this self-examination started, ask yourself the following questions.

• **How have the symptoms of arthritis affected my life?** It may be something simple: You no longer buy shoes with laces because it's too painful to tie them. Or it may be more complex: The fear that you can't handle more responsibility has kept you from seeking a job promotion.

• **How have others—my family, friends, coworkers, employer—been affected?** You may have noticed that those closest to you are going through the same feelings—anger, anxiety, denial, depression—that you are. At work, you may be avoiding certain tasks; if your colleagues or employer are unaware of your condition, they may see your behavior as laziness or lack of interest.

• **What feelings have I experienced lately?** Anger, sadness, depression are all understandable responses to realizing that your illness has changed you in some ways, has interfered with some of your goals or will be a constant concern for the rest of your life. How you react to or express these feelings can color how you manage your condition. For instance, your anger may lead you to defy your doctor or refuse medication; you may unconsciously direct your rage at family or friends—the people you now need most to give you support.

• **What is the biggest change in my life since symptoms began?** This change could be either a direct or indirect result of your arthritis: Perhaps you may have lost your job—or your interest in sex.

• **What has helped me to cope with my arthritis so far?** Has a phone call from a friend, listening to music or watching a funny movie distracted you from your pain? Perhaps at times you have found solace in your family or from your religion. By examining what has worked for you in the past, you and your doctor may be able to come up with several strategies you can rely on when you need them most.

As new concerns arise from your illness, try to confront them realistically and seek help before they become overwhelming. In some areas, you may be able to head off complications by preparing yourself, your family or others in your life for possible obstacles.

Effects . . . on Your Attitude

Arthritis may prey most heavily on your emotions, leaving you little psychic energy to cope with your condition. As discussed above, depression is a common reaction to having to deal daily with a chronic illness. It can discourage you from making the effort to feel better. It may lead you to withdraw, physically and emotionally, from family and friends. As you avoid certain situations and activities, your self-esteem may plummet. Self-confidence suffers too if you're no longer able to perform your usual tasks. At times you may wonder: Why bother?

You must remember that you need to keep in contact with those who care about you. Talk to them and teach them about your condition, so that they understand why you sometimes behave the way you do. Their support and encouragement will help lift your depression and spur you to comply with your treatment. Continue to pursue activities that you enjoy—even if you now can only be a spectator rather than a participant. Set new challenges for yourself too: Once you see how much you can accomplish, you'll be less likely to dwell on your limitations.

Chronic illness also means chronic stress. Even if you feel no discomfort right now, the specter of pain remains: When will it flare again? This anticipation can create physical as well as mental stress, as the body prepares itself to "fight or flee": Muscles tense, adrenaline courses through the blood, the heartbeat quickens. If this "emergency warning system" is activated often enough, you may feel exhausted, nervous and anxious nearly all the time.

Many of the techniques for managing pain, which are discussed in Chapter 6, are also effective for managing stress. Meditation, exercise, massage, biofeedback, even just talking about your struggles with a counselor or support group can relieve tension and allow you to cope during stressful periods. Understand, too, that if your life was already filled with stress—from financial or family problems, for example—your illness will only increase your anxiety, and in turn your anxiety may aggravate your illness. You may want to seek professional help to resolve these issues.

. . . In the Bedroom

Even though arthritis usually doesn't affect sexual function, it can easily inhibit your sex life. Pain, stiffness and fatigue in general will put a damper on your libido. Without doubt, if you have restricted movement in certain joints, such as the hips, you'll be physically limited in the way you perform. Remember, too, that some arthritis medications can depress your sex drive.

Your illness may also set up psychological barriers to making love. It may make you feel "old"—no longer a youthful, sexual being. If arthritis has deformed your joints, you may be self-conscious about your physical appearance. Your condition, and the other limitations it has imposed on you, may diminish your self-confidence in intimate relationships. If your partner seems afraid of causing you discomfort, your own pleasure may give way to concern for the other person's anxiety.

Too often these problems go unresolved because the topic causes embarrassment—for some doctors as well as patients. However, these difficulties can and should be dealt with, and you may have to make the first move

toward seeking advice. You may find that all you really
need is to plan ahead to minimize pain and maximize pleasure.

You may think that planning will take some of the
romance out of lovemaking, but it can have the opposite
effect. "Making a date" for sex with your partner can
create anticipation—an excitement that may make you
feel like a teenager again. Of course, you should set a time
when you know you'll be at your best. Be sure you're well
rested, and don't overtax yourself throughout the day.
Take your medication beforehand, when it will do the
most good. Soak in a warm bath, listen to music, light
scented candles or do anything else that relaxes you. We
hope that you've also been exercising regularly to preserve
your flexibility (see Chapter 5).

Still, the most important aspect of sexuality is commu-
nication with your partner. Be open—and open-minded—
when discussing your desires and concerns, and encourage
your partner to do the same. For instance, you may need
more time to relax and become aroused; your partner can
help through gentle massage or direct manual stimulation.
You may have to experiment to find the positions that are
most comfortable for you; the Arthritis Foundation's
booklet *Living and Loving* offers some suggestions.

If you've been able to discuss sexual matters before
arthritis became a problem, chances are that you'll continue to have a satisfying relationship despite the illness.
However, previous marital discord can only be heightened
by a chronic illness. You'll probably be wise to seek counseling to deal not only with this condition but with underlying issues. Your doctor should be able to help you find a
psychologist, social worker, therapist or other trained
counselor to guide you toward a better relationship.

Whatever happens, don't give up on this very vital aspect of your personal life. If you're past a certain age, you

may think you're too old to put much effort into enjoying sex, but it's more important now than ever. Intimacy and touch can soothe many ills. Sexual arousal stimulates the production of brain chemicals that can lift depression. It also triggers the release by the adrenal glands of cortisol, a natural arthritis-pain reliever for which you need no prescription!

... On Pregnancy

While most forms of arthritis don't directly affect your ability to become pregnant or deliver a healthy baby, you may have to consider your condition when deciding to have a child. About 75 percent of pregnant women with rheumatoid arthritis actually see some improvement: Joint swelling may lessen, though pain and stiffness may continue. Other arthritis conditions are less predictable; symptoms may get better, worsen or stay the same during the pregnancy. However, after the baby is born, your arthritis will probably flare. You may also feel worse for another reason: Because many drugs can harm a developing fetus, you'll probably be advised to stop taking some or all of your arthritis medications—even months before trying to conceive.

Not too long ago, women who had systemic lupus erythematosus were advised against giving birth, to prevent endangering their health and that of their offspring. Today many of the potential problems can be eliminated through careful monitoring and treatment during the pregnancy. Still, lupus patients are at the highest risk for complications. Your condition is likely to be aggravated somewhat during pregnancy and immediately after childbirth. If the disease has already affected your kidneys or heart, you may develop proteinuria (excess protein in the urine) or high blood pressure in pregnancy. Your condition may affect the growth of the fetus, which will be slower than normal. You have a greater chance than other expectant mothers of miscarriage, premature delivery and stillbirth; fortunately, doctors can test for substances in the blood that put you at higher risk for these complications. If you carry the antibody called anti-Ro or SSA, and perhaps another antibody, anti-La or SSB (both can also be detected by a blood test), your infant may develop heart block, a disorder that results in a slowed heartbeat. If the antigens HLA-DR3 and HLA-DR2 are present in your blood, you're more likely to deliver a child with neonatal lupus, the main feature of which is a skin rash that usually disappears within a year of birth. In general, lupus patients do best if they have been in remission six months before becoming pregnant.

Other arthritis sufferers, particularly those with rheumatoid arthritis, may develop carpal tunnel syndrome because of water retention constricting nerves in the wrists. (Actually, any pregnant woman can be afflicted by this condition, which can cause pain or numbness in the hands and fingers; it usually abates after childbirth.) If arthritis affects your hips or spine, your baby may have to be delivered by cesarean section, a surgical procedure that can involve a longer recovery time as well as postoperative complications such as infection or bleeding.

No matter what type of arthritis you have, you should also give careful consideration to the way your physical limitations will affect your caring for a child *after* it is born. In its first few years at least, you'll almost constantly be bending over, lifting and carrying your youngster. You'll have to be able to twist off the caps of baby-food jars and baby bottles, push a stroller, fasten tiny buttons or snaps. Also, you may not be able to breastfeed if you're on certain medications, which can be passed through your milk and be harmful to a baby. Remember too that ministering to an infant means less sleep—added fatigue that can worsen symptoms of your illness.

For any adult, not just the arthritis patient, raising a child is an awesome responsibility. Before deciding to become pregnant, talk to your doctor about any potential stumbling blocks. By taking precautions and planning ahead, you can minimize most risks to yourself and your baby.

. . . On the Job

Whether you're a construction worker or a clerk-typist, arthritis can present handicaps in the workplace. If you find that your condition is affecting your job performance—even before it becomes noticeable to your boss or coworkers—you should investigate your options. You can work with your doctor, who may refer you to a specialist such as an occupational therapist. You may discover that you can adapt equipment or your work space to ease difficulties; you can also consider switching to a more manageable position within the same company. Once you have some idea what you can do, discuss your situation with your employer or the firm's personnel director. Together you may come up with a plan that can keep you on the job.

The Rehabilitation Act of 1973 requires many businesses (those that deal with or receive funds from the federal government) to make provisions for handicaps, including arthritis. However, if your arthritis makes it impossible for you to continue with your present employer or to find other work, your local government can help. All fifty states and the District of Columbia support vocational rehabilitation programs, which can provide retraining, financial aid for education and other services that aim to get you back into the work force. You may also be able to make a claim on your disability insurance; contact your local Social Security Administration office.

. . . On Your Bank Account

Any chronic illness can be financially draining. Even the cost of a common over-the-counter anti-inflammatory drug like aspirin can add up when you're taking twelve or more tablets a day. Over the course of your illness, you may incur staggering expenses from monthly doctor visits, laboratory tests, medications, physical or occupational therapy, counseling, nursing care, homemaker services, canes or other mechanical aids, surgery, even transportation to and from appointments. No matter how comprehensive your health insurance, only some of these necessities or only a portion of their price tag may be covered. You should check with your carrier or your employee benefits office before running up any medical bill.

Ask your doctor to suggest ways to cut down costs—for instance, by ordering certain medications in larger quantities (this eliminates the fee you pay every time you fill a prescription at the pharmacy) or prescribing a generic drug instead of a brand name. Comparison-shop for your medications; prices can vary greatly from pharmacy to pharmacy. Mail-order drugs, available through agencies such as the American Association of Retired Persons, can be less expensive than store-bought medications. If you have already joined the Arthritis Foundation, take advantage of member discounts on drugs. Home health-care suppliers may sell used medical devices, such as canes, at lower cost. Sliding-scale fees, based on your ability to pay, may be arranged through county-funded counseling centers.

Depending on your circumstances, government assistance may also be available. You may be able to obtain short- or long-term disability benefits; check with your employer or local Social Security Administration office. You may also be eligible for Medicaid or Medicare, or financial aid from your state's Department of Social Service, or Welfare. Some help is also available for arthritis patients under age twenty-one through government programs such as your state's Crippled Children's Services.

When Your Child Has Arthritis

Childhood should be a relatively carefree time when all a youngster has to worry about is getting her homework done. When chronic illness afflicts a child, it can be overwhelming to her and her family. She should have an understanding of her condition, appropriate to her age. Be careful to explain why certain treatments are necessary and what they do; this information can ensure that she complies with doctor's orders. School personnel, such as teachers and nurses, should also be made aware of her medical requirements and restrictions.

Most children don't want to stand out or feel different, but having arthritis obviously sets a youngster apart from her peers. Thus the goal should be to maintain as normal a life for your child as possible; just keep plans flexible to allow for day-to-day changes in her health.

Expect your child to experience a range of emotions, including anger and self-pity. Encourage her to express these feelings and share some of your own, without burdening her with unnecessary worry. Show your concern for her but avoid the temptation to "make everything better"—taking over the child's chores or treating her like an invalid.

Your child may benefit most from learning she's not alone; seek out a support group where she can share her feelings with children who have the same or a similar condition. You and other family members also may find comfort and advice by talking to relatives of those with chronic illnesses. (The American Juvenile Arthritis Organization, a division of the Arthritis Foundation, may be able to connect you with such support groups; see "Specialized Organizations" in Chapter 12.)

In your concern for your affected child, don't neglect your own or your other children's needs and emotions. Parents may feel guilty, wondering whether something they did may have caused their youngster's arthritis. Siblings may also feel guilty if they begin to resent the attention to the other child. Explain to them as much as you can about their sibling's illness, and give them specific suggestions (not commands) on how they can help out. Stressing cooperation among family members will not only give the child a much-needed support system but will also make siblings feel that they're doing what they can to ease the suffering of a loved one.

In the chapters that follow, you'll learn about the treatments and techniques that will help you cope with these and other aspects of your arthritis.

CHAPTER 5

When to Exercise, When to Rest

The treatment program that you work out with your doctor may incorporate several strategies, including medication, pain management techniques and possibly surgery (these therapies are described in later chapters), and will take into account the type and severity of your arthritis. But for just about every arthritis sufferer, the one therapy that will do the most long-term good requires the most long-term commitment of time and attention: a well-thought-out plan of regular exercise.

Numerous studies have made it clear that the key to living well with arthritis is knowing when to be active, when to protect your joints from undue stress and when to rest them. Finding and maintaining this delicate balance between exercise and rest are ultimately up to you. You must be diligent in following your regimen and plan how to fit it into your everyday routine; you must always be aware of your own physical condition and when to conserve your energy. There may be days—many days—when the last thing you want to do is lace up your walking shoes and head out for a stroll around the block. At other times, you'll want to do more than your body will allow. Knowing when you can ignore some signals and when you can give in to others is a process of trial and error. Don't give up! The benefits are well worth your effort.

Exercising Your Options

If right now arthritis pain is a daily companion, you may wonder how you can bring yourself to exercise at all. Your instinct may be to move your joints as little as possible and to avoid any activity beyond the minimum. But you must believe that getting up and around is necessary to maintaining and even improving whatever joint function you now have. The sooner you get started, the better, to head off any future damage.

Not too long ago, doctors ordered inactivity or complete bed rest for patients with arthritis—a prescription we now know would worsen many forms of the disease. Restricting movement further limits a joint's range of motion—the extent to which it can naturally move in any direction. In extreme cases, unused joints can fuse, or can lock into a bent position, a condition called *flexion contracture*. So the updated advice for an arthritis sufferer is: Use it or lose it!

Besides the disservice to your joints, a sedentary life dooms you to even more health problems. Neglected muscles can weaken, losing up to 3 percent of their function per day, according to a 1966 study published in the *Journal of the American Medical Association*. This makes you more vulnerable to all types of injury. Bones too need to be stressed in order to maintain their density; otherwise, they can become fragile and fracture easily—a disorder known as osteoporosis.

For the arthritis patient, exercise can go a long way

toward improving joints: With regular activity, you'll enjoy greater flexibility and suffer less pain. Other benefits may indirectly influence your arthritis: You'll feel less fatigued, have increased energy and be more fit overall. You'll have greater endurance. Exercise stimulates the release of endorphins from the brain; these "feel-good" chemicals help banish depression. As you reach your fitness goals, you're bound to feel a renewed self-confidence along with a sense of accomplishment—a great boon to your spirit!

Not all forms of activity bring about the same results, and some might be off-limits to you because of the joints involved. Your exercise program must be tailored to you with your doctor's guidance; he or she will probably have you consult or work with a physical therapist (PT) or occupational therapist (OT). (The jobs of these two types of licensed professionals can vary from one health-care facility to the next. In general, though, a PT can teach you the various therapeutic exercises and certain pain relief techniques, such as the hot and cold treatments that are described in Chapter 6. An OT can show you how to plan and perform tasks at home or at work more efficiently, how to adapt your living areas to your best advantage, and how to use splints, canes and other assistive devices.) The following will give you a general idea of the exercises you may be prescribed and how they'll help you.

Types of Exercise

For the majority of arthritis patients, a *therapeutic program* will be designed to target affected tissues and offset other possible complications of the disease. Even if your condition requires joint surgery, physical therapy will help you to recover after the operation and to maintain joint function for the rest of your life. You will most likely be advised to include three categories of exercise: range of motion, strengthening, and endurance.

Range of Motion

This type of exercise involves gently stretching the muscles surrounding the affected joints, to prevent the muscles, ligaments and tendons from pulling the joint into a bent or deformed position and tightening permanently. Series of exercises for each body part are designed to move a joint through all its possible directions. The intensity can vary according to your condition and how much inflammation you may be experiencing on a particular day.

The benefits from this type of exercise can be enormous for those with arthritis. It can maintain and even improve the directions in which you can move pain-free. It can restore flexibility to the joint, making movement easier. In addition, it can relieve your stiffness throughout the day.

Following is one range of motion exercise for the hips. In this example, you lie on the floor with legs about ten inches apart and toes pointing up. Then roll your entire leg (one at a time) inward and outward, without bending your knee. Repeat five to ten times.

For finger flexibility, there are many variations on the movement following. Here, you try to touch each finger to the tip of your thumb to form an O, spreading out your five fingers wide after each touch. Repeat five to ten times. To add some resistance, twist a rubber band among all the fingers of the hand.

Exercises such as these should be begun as soon as possible, as a daily part of arthritis treatment. Even if you're bedridden, you can be assisted—by a loved one, physical

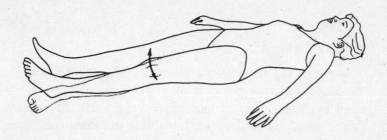

RANGE OF MOTION EXERCISE FOR HIPS

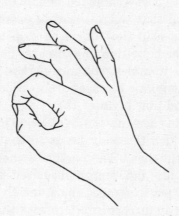

FLEXIBILITY EXERCISE
FOR FINGERS

therapist or occupational therapist—through these motions. (If you're severely disabled, someone can be instructed and properly trained to move your joints for you; this is called passive exercise.)

Strengthening

Because the muscles stabilize and support the joints, keeping them strong is crucial. If your muscles are weakened by disuse, you cannot move your joint through its full range of motion. Strength training becomes even more important as you age, because muscles naturally shrink each year after your twenties. You remain strong only if you tax your muscles regularly. If you avoid much strenuous activity because of your arthritis, you're losing muscle strength at an even faster rate. Those with rheumatoid arthritis, for instance, have about 60 percent less muscle strength than that of unaffected people of the same age.

Keep in mind that weight-bearing exercise also builds bone. That can help slow down or stop the progress of osteoporosis, the bone-thinning disease that afflicts many people, especially women past menopause. Those with inflammatory rheumatic diseases are particularly susceptible to this condition because they often are inactive or rarely get out in the sun. (Sunlight helps form vitamin D on the skin, which the body needs so that it can absorb calcium from the diet.) Some arthritis medications, such as corticosteroids and aluminum-based antacids (they may be prescribed to protect the stomach from other arthritis drugs), can further interfere with the absorption of calcium.

One type of strength training that can be performed by nearly every person with arthritis is *isometric exercise:* It involves little or no movement of the joint itself, because the muscle force is applied against an immovable object or body part. For instance, to build up your arms, you can stand in a doorway and push against the door frame with your hands (see illustration below), holding the muscle contraction for about six to ten seconds; relax, then repeat, for a total of five times. Simply pressing your hands or thighs together as hard as you can is also an isometric exercise. Isometrics have some limitations: They don't build strength through a muscle's full range of motion; they also increase blood pressure, so are a poor choice for those who also have hypertension or heart disease. Generally, though, isometrics are simple, safe moves that require no special equipment or workout space.

Isotonic exercises are what most people associate with

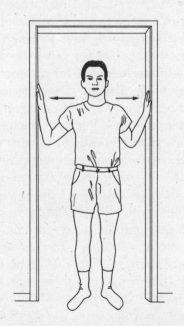

ISOMETRIC EXERCISE

building muscles: For these, a load, such as a movable weight or the weight of your own body, provides the resistance as the muscles contract to raise and lower it. Exercises can include calisthenics like sit-ups or push-ups, weight lifting with dumbbells or barbells, and working out with a resistance machine such as the Eagle, Nautilus or Universal system, or with special color-coded rubber exercise bands. Besides giving greater gains in strength and endurance (the ability of the muscle to sustain an activity) than isometrics, isotonic activities are able to work a joint and muscle through its entire range of motion. However, too many repetitions with too heavy a weight can aggravate inflammation. Also, if full movement is painful for your joints, you may not be able to perform the exercises.

Ronald Cahn, physical therapist at the Hospital for Joint Diseases, suggests that alternating isometric with isotonic exercises can be the key to maintaining a well-balanced strengthening program: During flares, try submaximum isometrics, since they put little stress on joints; during less painful periods, opt for an isotonic workout.

To maintain basic fitness, the American College of Sports Medicine currently recommends strength training at least two times a week. (Very strenuous exercises for a particular muscle group should not be performed two days in a row; muscles need about forty-eight hours to recover from a workout.) Of course, how often and how long you train must be decided with the help of your doctor and physical therapist, who will evaluate you on the basis of your age, physical capabilities, symptoms, overall health and other risk factors. It's best, too, to develop not only the muscles supporting an affected joint but all muscle groups equally; one area that is weaker than others is vulnerable to injury. Don't attempt to begin a strength training program on your own; a physical therapist should instruct you on how to do the exercises properly and may require that you be supervised.

If you think it's too late for you to take up weight lifting, you haven't heard about a recent study from Tufts University. When a group of nursing home residents were supervised in an eight-week weight training program, the formerly frail ninety-year-olds showed a remarkable increase in muscle size; they improved their mobility so much that some were able to put aside their walkers for the first time in many years!

Endurance

This is what you get from aerobics—exercises that pump the heart and lungs, forcing you take in extra oxygen to be carried through the blood to the muscles. Heavy-breathing activities not only strengthen the cardiovascular system, they also require that the body pull out and burn its stored fat. In a nutshell: Regular aerobic activity can lower blood pressure, aid in weight loss, boost energy, lessen stress and reduce your risk for heart disease, diabetes and some cancers—eliminating the other health problems that often befall sedentary people with arthritis. It will also improve some muscle tone and range of motion. Who can argue with that kind of success?

The type of aerobic exercise you should choose hinges on your condition and the joints involved. Generally, unless you have major knee pain, you can get going with walking and biking (stationary cycling is even safer and more convenient). Cross-country skiing causes fewer injuries and is more aerobic than downhill skiing; sliding forward on snow is less stressful on lower joints, while working the ski poles builds the upper body. Dancing and rowing are other aerobic options. But swimming is probably number one for those who have arthritis: Since the water buoys up your body, there's no pressure on joints. If you can work out in a heated pool, so much the better; the warmth can soothe your aches while you do laps. Even if you can't swim, you can try aquatic exercises; simple moves like leg lifts or walking have an added advantage in the water, which supplies about twelve times the resistance of air.

Aerobic exercise that is jarring to affected joints should be avoided. Hip, knee or back problems, for instance, would rule out jogging, high-impact aerobic dance, rope-jumping or stair-stepping. Before beginning *any* aerobic exercise program, you should be medically cleared by your physician.

In order for an aerobic activity to boost cardiovascular fitness, the American College of Sports Medicine suggests that it be performed for at least twenty minutes, three or more days per week. In addition, that twenty minutes should be at an intensity called the training heart rate. This is calculated by subtracting your age from 220 (the maximum heart rate), then multiplying that number by 60 and 80 percent to get an acceptable range. For example, if you're fifty-five, your target heart rate zone is 99 to 132 heartbeats per minute ($220 - 55 = 165 \times .6$ and $.8$). Then, the next time you exercise, take your pulse and count the number of heartbeats in six seconds and multiply by ten to see if you're within that range. This intensity may not be advisable for some arthritis patients. Others may not be able to exercise long enough or hard enough to reach the target zone at first, but will get there if they stay faithful to their program.

Any *recreational activity* that you enjoy and that helps you relax should also be incorporated into your fitness schedule. Sports like golf or bowling, hobbies like bird-watching or gardening, crafts like quilting or woodworking won't improve your joint function nearly as much as the therapeutic exercises, but added to that regimen, they may better your range of motion and muscle strength, and they're certainly beneficial for overall health of body and mind. Some recreational sports like baseball, which provides little aerobic benefit and whose twist-and-turn moves can injure joints, should be resumed only after you're in better shape from your therapeutic program.

Everyday activities, too, can keep you limber. Getting washed and dressed, combing your hair, cleaning the house, preparing meals, climbing stairs or mowing the lawn may take an effort, but every little bit helps to tone muscles. Many patients benefit from instruction by an occupational therapist to maximize their ability to perform their activities of daily living. These activities also keep you connected to the daily routine you had before arthritis struck—a benefit to your peace of mind. But again, because these tasks don't often use a joint's full range of motion, they're no substitute for a regular program of therapeutic exercise.

Getting Started

- Before beginning any exercise program, get your doctor's approval.
- Start slowly, gradually increasing the time and intensity of your exercise. Movements should be smooth and slow, while you breathe deeply and rhythmically.
- Apply a hot compress or take a warm shower or bath for about twenty minutes before your activity, to ease inflammation and relax joints and muscles.
- Always warm up before and cool down after exercise, for about five to ten minutes. That means performing

a slowed-down version of the activity. For example, stroll before you begin a brisk walk, then gradually decrease your pace to finish up.

- Stretch slowly and gently for a few minutes before, but even more importantly after, any strengthening or aerobic exercise to limber up muscles and tendons (exercise will tighten them).

- To help you stick to an aerobic program, choose an activity that you enjoy but that is convenient for you too. For instance, you may love to swim, but if you have to drive across town to get to a pool, you probably won't do it very often. Walking in your neighborhood or riding a stationary bike in your bedroom may be easier for you to manage most days. Or plan an alternative or rainy-day activity for when you can't manage your first choice.

- Listen to your body. If a joint is inflamed, move it very gently through its range of motion. Take advantage of less painful periods by stepping up activity. During flare-ups, reduce your efforts.

- If a particular exercise is causing you difficulty, let your doctor know. The doctor or your physical therapist may be able to modify it so that it will be easier for you.

- Learn how to perform an exercise properly. Incorrect positioning or form can add insult to an injured joint.

- Pick a partner. Working out with a companion or in a group can help keep you motivated and encouraged.

- Dress for success. Comfortable clothes—loose, lightweight—will give you freedom of movement; wear layers so that you can add or subtract clothing as you heat up or cool down. Wear clothes with snaps or large buttons if your hands are affected.

- Wear appropriate footgear for the activity. For example, walking shoes are great for a stroll because they're well cushioned at the heels, but for low-impact aerobics, they won't give support where you need it—at the ball of the foot. Instead, they'll trip you up and you may be sidelined by injury. If you have a specific problem like overpronation (your feet "roll in" too much, which can put a strain on knees or hips), you may benefit from orthopodics. These custom-fitted shoe inserts can correct many foot imbalances and misalignments; a podiatrist or orthopedist can prescribe a pair for you.

- Set goals for yourself, and keep a log of your progress. Seeing how far you've come will spur you to keep up the good work.
- Find the time of day when it's least tiring for you to exercise. You may discover that early activity helps your morning stiffness, or that you don't feel energetic until the afternoon.
- Schedule your workout to coincide with the time your medication is most effective.
- Stop exercising if you notice severe or unusual pain—in your joints or in any other part of your body, such as the chest. Dizziness, nausea, difficulty breathing and faintness are other signs of trouble. Don't ignore them!

Conserving Your Energy

Too much exercise can be as harmful to your joints as too little, furthering inflammation and damage. If pain persists two hours past performing any activity, you may need to cut down on how long or how hard you're doing it.

Certainly a flare-up should be a signal to ease back. But rather than giving yourself over to complete inactivity, schedule regular rest periods. They'll renew your strength as well as reduce pain, inflammation and even psychological stress. To be sure that you don't overdo it and that you get the most out of every day, follow the three P's of time management:

• **Plan** ahead. If you think about what you have to do well before you do it, you can figure out ways to simplify the task or take shortcuts. Organize your errands so you won't be bounding from one end of the house—or one end of town—to the other in one day. Organize your work areas—in the kitchen, in your basement, on the job—to minimize your efforts and to keep equipment within easy reach.

• **Pace** yourself. Tackle a project far enough in advance so that you can do a bit each day (for instance, painting a room) or over several hours (preparing dinner). Avoid doing two strenuous activities in a row. Alternate standing tasks with chores you can manage sitting down. And sandwich busy periods between rest stops.

• **Prioritize** your tasks. Each day or the night before, make a list of what you want to accomplish, from the most to the least important. If you don't get to the last item or two, don't sweat it: You've already done what you most needed to do. You may also find that many of the chores you set up for yourself are not really necessary or can be done less often.

Also keep in mind a fourth P: *Plead*. Don't hesitate to ask for a hand from your family, friends or coworkers if you can't finish a project, reach a high shelf, move a bulky object. Often we let pride get in the way of doing what is in our own best interests. In truth, most people like to feel needed and will be happy to help; if you can, rotate your requests so that the same person isn't always called upon. Certainly delegate more tasks to other family members, even if those chores have "traditionally" been yours; if your relatives are made aware of your limitations in a direct manner, they'll *want* to pitch in.

Here are a few more suggestions for giving your joints a break. Your physician, a physical therapist or an occupational therapist can offer other guidelines for specific problems you may be experiencing.

In general:

• Avoid fatigue. This means ensuring a good night's sleep by getting to bed early before a busy day, or refusing to worry about circumstances over which you have no control.

• If your knees are painful, choose chairs with armrests. You'll be able to stand up more easily by pushing your open palms against the chair arms, putting less weight on your knees.

• Don't bend or twist your joints unnecessarily by wriggling with your hips to get out of a chair, for example, or reaching from an awkward position.

• Rely on the larger muscle groups and the strongest joints. For instance, push rather than pull with muscles. Push open a door with your shoulder or hip rather than your hand. Untwist a jar lid with your full palm rather than your bent fingers.

• When climbing stairs, set the same foot forward each time, bringing the other foot next to it on the stair. Lead with your stronger leg on the way up; on the way down, step first with your weaker leg.

• Distribute the weight of an object over several joints. For instance, grasp a glass or mug in both hands. Place both palms on the bottom of an object to lift or

hold it, instead of gripping it with your fingers. Carry packages with both hands, close to your body.
* Whenever possible, sit while working.
* To prevent stiffness, shift your position often.
* Avoid doing too much—even on a "good" day—or your "bad" days may return that much sooner!

Around the house:

* Transport cleaning supplies, linens and laundry from room to room in a wheeled cart or table.
* Use long-handled, lightweight cleaning implements to avoid bending and reaching. You can buy extenders or attach dowels to existing handles.
* Use swan-neck shovels, rakes and other tools, which require less bending.
* Wear an apron with many pockets to carry supplies and keep them at hand.
* Install lazy Susans or pull-out shelves for easier access to cabinet space.
* Store heavy items at waist height.
* Place a rubber pad under containers to keep them from slipping as you open them. Another pad or rubber gloves can help you twist off tight lids.

In the kitchen:

* Consider buying adaptive equipment to help you with certain tasks. For instance, grocery-store-type reachers can help you pull down items from the back of cabinets or high shelves.
* Choose utensils with wide or gripper handles. You can also build up handles yourself by slipping on thick, lightweight tubing (such as a foam hair curler, a rubber bicycle-handlebar grip or pipe insulation) or wrapping a piece of padding around the handle.

- Choose lightweight cookware (aluminum) and dinner-ware (plastic).
- Use nonstick cookware, which takes less effort to clean.
- Use appliances—an electric knife, dishwasher, can opener, mixer, blender or food processor—to cut down on the use of finger joints.
- Buy long tongs to let you flip food in the oven or broiler without having to lean over too far.
- If you have trouble bending your neck or gripping a glass, drink from a straw.
- If your fingers ache from gripping, slip on oven mitts for moving hot food or a sponge mitt for washing dishes.
- Keep a step stool handy for sitting while cooking or washing, and for reaching high shelves.

In the bathroom:

- Have handrails installed in the tub and near the toilet.
- Place a plastic seat or a transfer bench in the tub so that you can sit while showering.
- Use nonslip (rubber-backed) mats inside and outside the tub.
- Think about buying an electric toothbrush, which has a thicker, easier-to-grip handle and requires less arm movement. If this device is too heavy for you, build up your toothbrush handle with foam padding.
- Use a long-handled bristle or sponge brush to scrub your back and other hard-to-reach spots.
- Organize a tub tray or shower caddy to keep shampoo, soap and other toiletries at hand.
- Use a detachable, hand-held showerhead so you can rinse off easily or wash while sitting.
- Replace faucet controls with lever-type handles,

which can be moved with your palms rather than grasped with your fingers.
- Buy toothpaste in a pump dispenser.

In the bedroom:

- Choose the best-quality mattress you can afford. It's worth it for a good night's sleep. Firm is usually better for supporting ailing joints.
- Have the bed raised. You'll be able to make the bed while sitting, and get out of it more easily.
- Buy fitted bottom sheets, one size bigger than your bed, to eliminate tucking and slip easily over corners.
- Tuck in sheets with a wooden paddle or pancake turner to save stress on arthritic fingers.
- Attach rails to the side of the bed so that you can pull yourself up to sit or stand.
- Add a ring or chain to zipper tabs on clothing to make them easier to zip up.
- Choose slip-on shoes or those that fasten with Velcro. A shoemaker can adapt your current footwear, putting in a Velcro closure instead of a buckle.
- Wear clip-on neckties.

In the workshop:

- Choose cordless electric tools like screwdrivers and drills.
- Carry tools from project to project in a tool belt or carpenter's apron.
- Transport heavy items on a hand truck or wheelbarrow.
- Wrap tool handles with cushioned tape to build them up and give a nonslip grip.
- If you need to keep a steady hold on pliers, use a locking pair.

- Set up a small storage cabinet or pegboard for holding tools near your workbench.

In the office:

- Use a pencil to dial a rotary phone or to push the buttons on a Touch-tone phone.
- Build up pencil or pen shafts with a slip-on foam hair curler.
- Use felt-tip pens, which allow lighter finger pressure.
- Be sure work surfaces and chairs are at a comfortable height.
- Try electric scissors or a battery-powered letter opener.
- Set papers in an adjustable book stand so that you can read without straining your neck.

At your leisure:

- Slot playing cards into the bristles of an upturned scrub brush so that you don't tire holding them.
- Place a lazy Susan under a checkers or Scrabble gameboard so that you can revolve it and not have to reach so far when it's your turn.
- Check gardening catalogs for a lightweight bench with side grips, to sit or kneel on while you're working in the garden.
- When traveling, take along a horseshoe-shaped pillow to cushion your neck and head.
- Use a padded cloth steering-wheel cover to allow a looser grip for your fingers; the surface will never get too hot or too cold to touch.
- Schedule shopping or other outings for midweek or off-peak times, when you'll be less likely to have to battle crowds or stand on long lines.

• Do your packing in lightweight, wheeled luggage. Drape bags with shoulder straps across your body to distribute weight and leave your hands free.

Mechanical Aids

If your knees, hips, back or feet make walking painful, your doctor may suggest you use a gait aid—a cane, crutches, walker or wheelchair—to take the weight off these joints. (Your physical therapist will need to assess you and train you in using it.) You may find you need to use such an aid only at certain times. For instance, when traveling by plane, take advantage of the wheelchairs available from airlines to transport passengers to the flight gate. Why waste energy that can otherwise be spent more enjoyably at your destination?

A splint—or sometimes a brace or cast—may also be recommended by your physician, physical therapist or occupational therapist. The rigid support can be strapped to a joint, such as the wrist or knee, at night or during the day, either to rest it, protect it or prevent it from contracting into a bent position. Don't use a splint without a doctor's or therapist's supervision; if it's not chosen, fitted and monitored carefully, a splint can further deform or weaken joints.

Many other aids are also available that make everyday tasks easier on your joints: They'll help you zip up zippers, open car doors, sew on a button, and much more. In its *Guide to Independent Living*, the Arthritis Foundation has compiled hundreds of mail-order sources for such items (see "Exercise and Joint Protection" in Chapter 12).

As a general precaution, protective devices cannot be substituted for exercise. Without some type of regular activity, muscles will weaken and joints will stiffen to a point beyond rehabilitation. Follow your doctor's orders regarding when protection would be appropriate, and if you have any questions about using a particular aid, talk to your physician or therapist.

CHAPTER 6

Managing Pain

Dull or sharp, fleeting or constant—pain is the most common and disruptive aspect of arthritis. As an arthritis patient, you'll most likely be living daily with the threat as well as the reality of pain: Even when you're feeling well, you may be anticipating your next flare.

Your doctor may prescribe medications to fight inflammation and ease pain; in more extreme cases, surgery may offer the only relief. Yet surgery is often a last resort, and drugs have their own dangers when relied on too frequently or for the long term (these issues are explored in Chapters 7 and 8). As discussed in Chapter 5, exercise and rest can help reduce or eliminate painful episodes. This chapter offers other nonmedicinal therapies that will help you handle the chronic stress and distress of pain. Your goal should be to control your pain instead of letting it control you.

And you can. Pain is unpredictable but manageable; it's difficult to define, explain or measure, but it has certain identifiable features. For instance, dwelling on it can intensify it; distracting from it can make it "go away." How much pain you feel and when you feel it often hinge on your personal pain tolerance: Everyone has his or her own threshold—the level at which the merely annoying becomes excruciating. Many factors—your emotions, attitude, lifestyle—can raise or lower this threshold.

Using noninvasive physical and mental techniques, you can block or cut back on your discomfort. To see how this is possible, you need to understand the mechanisms involved in the sensation we call "pain."

The Nature of Pain

Pain is the body's warning system. Nerve endings near the injured site are stimulated, sending impulses to other nerves along the spinal cord, then to the brain. For arthritis sufferers, this pain "telegraph" is triggered by chemicals released during the inflammation process that act on nerves. Other nerve-stimulating substances are produced when cartilage or bone is damaged, or when muscles become strained.

Though these pathways of pain are universal, research has shown that the message is received differently by different people and at different times, depending on each person's physical and mental states. Many scientists believe we all have a "pain gate"—a mechanism located in the spinal column that allows pain to reach the brain. This gate can be opened by stress, fatigue or focusing on the discomfort; luckily, these are factors over which we have some control. Also, because our nervous system can only process so much information at a time, we can close this gate ourselves by activating other stimuli that shut out the pain. For instance, most people—and animals too—unconsciously attempt to soothe a sore spot by rubbing it.

This self-massage sends a pleasant message instead of the painful one: Like all enjoyable sensations, it stimulates the release of endorphins, brain chemicals that enhance pleasure and interrupt the transmission of the pain message. In arthritis treatment, applying heat or cold to a joint, stretching muscles or even cultivating a positive outlook can provide the stimulation that cancels out pain.

When you're tired or sad, you can't summon up the physical or mental energy to close the pain gate. Muscles become tense, causing greater anguish. If your situation seems helpless or hopeless, you become increasingly discouraged. Pain creates stress, which leads to depression, which worsens pain, which creates stress, which . . . You get the picture. Discovering ways to close the pain gate can put an end to this unhealthy cycle.

Taking Charge

Taking charge of pain means making changes: in the way you view your arthritis and yourself. Of course, your nervous system may be so sensitive or your illness so severe that pain is unavoidable. But to some extent you can alter your response to pain, especially if it was a learned behavior from your past or is a result of circumstances in the present.

For instance, some people are "taught" how to perceive pain in their childhood: If your parents bandaged your scrapes and then sent you back out to play, you're more likely to deal with a setback matter-of-factly, then move on. On the other hand, if you were fussed over or sent to bed whenever you were hurt, you might be self-pitying or passive in the face of pain.

For other people, the degree of pain may relate to their

current situation: You may be overworked, feel neglected by your spouse or children, feel overwhelmed by money worries or afraid of losing your job. When you're suffering distress in one area of your life, it will magnify whatever pain your arthritis causes.

The strategies that follow for managing pain offer a wide range of approaches. From them, you can put together your own "first-aid kit." Some may work better for you than others or may succeed only in certain circumstances; some may lose their effectiveness over time. These suggestions may also trigger ideas of your own.

Change Your Attitude

Even Hamlet, who spent much of Shakespeare's play brooding on his troubles, said, "There is nothing either good or bad, but thinking makes it so." Readjusting your mental outlook can often make the difference between good and bad days.

• **Don't dwell on it.** (That was Hamlet's undoing.) Arthritis patients who focus too much attention on their pain report much more intense symptoms. If pain occupies your thoughts, evict it with more productive mental processes, such as learning a new language via cassette tapes or working a crossword puzzle. Take your mind off your pain by watching a funny movie, calling a friend or listening to music.

Keep a list of tried-and-true distractions.

• **Accentuate the positive.** Medical science has confirmed the power of positive thinking: Having pleasant thoughts actually changes your brain chemistry. Even if you force yourself to smile when feeling glum, your mind will gradually shift to match your expression. So when pain hits, think of the pluses in your life: Your grandchildren, good friends, a satisfying career or hobby. Then use this positive energy to convince yourself you can cope with your arthritis: "I *can* feel better by continuing my stretching exercises." When you find yourself thinking "I can't," substitute a statement that begins with "I can."

• **Meditate.** This Eastern discipline controls concentration, blocking out pain signals. You can be instructed in transcendental meditation, or try it yourself by repeating (out loud or in your head) a simple sound or phrase, such as "Om" or "I can." You can get the same effect by visualizing a single, soothing image (such as a tranquil lake) or by focusing on breathing, slowly and evenly, from your abdomen. Perform such exercises for at least twenty minutes while sitting in a comfortable, quiet spot.

• **Talk to others.** Join an arthritis support group to share your feelings and frustrations about your condition with others, outside of your family, who have the same concerns. Besides releasing anger and reducing depression, you'll pick up ideas for coping, some inspirational stories and a new friend or two. Having sympathetic listeners is sure to boost your spirits and lessen the pain. Your doctor or local Arthritis Foundation chapter can recommend a support group for you—and for your family.

• **Seek counseling.** If your pain or other personal concerns are so overwhelming that you can't seem to cope with your illness, you may need a psychotherapist to guide you. Don't be afraid to ask for this kind of help;

it's a sensible, courageous step toward living with a chronic problem. A psychiatrist, psychologist or psychiatric social worker may be available to you through your health-care facility, or you can ask your doctor for a referral.

Another option is a pain clinic. These centers are usually staffed with a variety of health-care professionals, including psychiatrists, rehabilitation doctors, psychologists, rheumatologists, anesthesiologists, neurologists, physical and occupational therapists, vocational counselors and social workers. Such a facility may be able to offer you more personalized, intensive and comprehensive care in pain management. Your doctor, local rehabilitation hospital or medical school, or the American Pain Society (see "Pain Management" in Chapter 12) can help you find a pain center near you.

Change Your Behavior

You may have an unhealthy lifestyle or personal habits—developed before or after the onset of your arthritis—that could be contributing to your pain. Vow to do only what's good for you.

• **Eat properly.** When in pain, you may bypass well-balanced meals for high-fat, high-calorie snacks as a way to comfort yourself—or you may not feel like eating at all. As is discussed in Chapter 9, poor diet can cause physical and mental fatigue that makes it difficult to cope with arthritis pain.

• **Sleep well.** The most common complaint of chronic-pain sufferers is loss of sleep, and the resulting fatigue only aggravates pain. Do all you can to ensure a good night's rest. Time your medication so that it will be working while you try to fall asleep. Avoid stimulants like tobacco and caffeine, especially after midafternoon. (Caffeine can be found not only in coffee, tea and colas, but also in cocoa and other chocolate products, some herbal teas and noncola soft drinks such as Mountain Dew and Dr Pepper. It's also an unsuspected ingredient in many nonprescription pharmaceuticals which combine caffeine and medicines, such as certain brands of weight-loss aids, aspirin, acetaminophen, menstrual-pain relievers, antihistamines, decongestants, and alertness aids; check to see whether the product's label lists caffeine or ask your pharmacist.)

Engaging in an aerobic exercise several hours before bedtime can help you sleep—not only because it tires you out, but because it raises your body temperature. Body temperature naturally falls as you fall asleep; when your temperature is higher from exercise, the drop is greater, leading to deeper, better sleep. Work out about three to four hours before bedtime: If earlier, you won't reap the benefit; if later, you may be too wound up to drop off.

If your nighttime sleep is disturbed, sneak in a nap or two during the day for at least twenty minutes. You'll feel more refreshed and able to deal with whatever comes your way.

• **Exercise.** As you learned in the previous chapter, proper stretching exercises can ward off or reduce painful episodes. You also know that sustained aerobic activity triggers the release of those painkilling endorphins. Exercise can help you relax by relieving physical tension, and (as mentioned above) can help you sleep. In addition, overall fitness reduces the risk of diseases that can contribute to pain.

• **Have fun.** Leisure pursuits will keep you mentally and physically active—which is necessary to counteract pain. Even if you can't participate, spectate.

• **Socialize.** Contact with others not only distracts you from your pain, it's psychologically soothing. Besides visiting with family and friends, do volunteer work, take an adult-education class, or join a hobby club to motivate you to get out and about.

• **Relax.** Tension intensifies pain, so try to banish unnecessary stresses from your life. When you can't sidestep an aggravating situation, consciously try to control and calm yourself. You might use meditation, deep breathing or visualization, as described above. Yoga is the perfect tranquilizer for arthritis sufferers, as it combines stretching exercises with focused breathing. You can also practice progressive relaxation techniques, such as deliberately tensing, then releasing particular muscle groups one at a time; or repeating spoken commands to relax each body part (for example: "My right arm feels heavy and warm").

• **Avoid drug dependence.** If you try to escape by using alcohol or illegal drugs or overusing the medications prescribed for your arthritis, you will do damage to your body and add to your pain. Let healthy habits take their place.

Learn Self-Help Treatments

These pain management methods should be begun only after consulting with your doctor, who may need to instruct you or monitor you in their use. Some can be dangerous if overused or performed incorrectly.

• **Thermotherapy.** Heat can ease pain, raise your pain threshold, relax muscle spasms and relieve joint stiffness. There are many ways to apply warmth to an aching area (also see "Diathermy" below). The following are superficial treatments, meaning that they don't penetrate far below the skin surface, but are still effective for less severe joint pain.

A *hot shower,* a *warm bath* or short stay in a *sauna* can soothe your whole body. A *hot-water bottle* wrapped in a towel can be placed on a painful joint. Some prefer the moist heat of a *hot compress*—a cloth soaked in hot water, then wrung out. *Hot packs,* filled with a heat-retaining gel, are also available. A *heating pad* or a *heat lamp* can be used at a low setting, but be sure you're alert; falling asleep under one can cause burns. For morning stiffness, try an *electric blanket* or *mattress pad,* but the same cautions apply: Be careful not to set the thermostat too high or doze off while using it.

Some people dip their hands in a *paraffin bath*—a mixture of melted wax and mineral oil. The coating stays warmer longer and doesn't dry out your skin, but otherwise has no other advantage over a warm-water soak. Don't use this method if you have cuts or other open wounds on your hands.

Deep-heat lotions, some having a numbing effect and others creating a warm tingling sensation, can be rubbed on your skin. Never use these rubs with a heating pad or other heat application: This can cause the ointment to penetrate too far into your skin and damage underlying tissues.

Which heat method you choose will have more to do with where your pain is located than how well each works. For instance, your hand would be more evenly warmed by immersing it in heated water; your neck and shoulders can more easily be treated with a hot pack.

Surface heat should be applied for no longer than twenty minutes, as it may actually increase swelling or result in scalding. You can repeat treatments throughout the day, but wait at least thirty minutes between applications. If you have poor blood circulation or numbness in the affected area, you should not use heat treatments. In the first case, your cardiovascular system may not be efficient enough to help your body release the excess heat; in the other, you may not be able to tell if the treatment is burning your skin.

• **Cryotherapy.** Cold can help numb painful tissue by slowing down nerve activity; it also will reduce swelling. You can massage a small area with an ice cube for one to two minutes. Larger areas can be treated with a cold pack (a silicate-gel-filled plastic bag)—or, in an emergency, a bag of ice or frozen food. A cold compress can also be made by dipping a cloth in ice water, then wringing it out before placing it on the joint. Coolant sprays, like those sold for sunburn, can also provide spot relief.

You can apply cold for fifteen to twenty minutes, three to four times a day. As with heat treatments, don't apply any cold pack or ice cube to bare skin; wrap it in a cloth or thin towel first.

• **Contrast baths.** Applying both hot and cold in one treatment brings relief to some arthritis sufferers. Hands or feet can be soaked first in a basin of hot water (about 110 degrees Fahrenheit) for three minutes, then in one of cold (about 65 degrees) for one minute.

• **Hydrotherapy.** Water can soothe in several ways: If you immerse yourself in it, it will buoy you up, taking pressure off joints; if heated, it relaxes muscles; if moving, it provides a gentle massage. If you have a whirlpool or a Jacuzzi at your disposal, so much the better. A Hubbard tank—a heated tub that allows total immersion—may be available through your physical therapist but should be used under supervision. Also, as mentioned in Chapter 5, you'll find that you can perform your range of motion exercises more easily in warmed water.

• **Diathermy.** For this deep-heating treatment, special equipment generates heat energy by shortwave (high-frequency radio waves), microwave (high-frequency electromagnetic waves) or ultrasound (high-frequency sound waves). Shortwave won't penetrate deep enough to reach joints such as the hip and is chiefly used to ease muscle spasms. Microwave cannot treat the bonier areas like elbows and cannot be used near metallic surgical implants. Ultrasound is often the best all-around choice: It reaches deepest, its sound waves agitate molecules to create heat within joints, and it can be used safely with implants.

All forms of diathermy should be avoided if the affected area has poor circulation, reduced sensation, or severe inflammation or swelling. Patients with pacemakers should not be treated with shortwave or microwave.

• **Massage.** Performed either by you or by a partner, gentle rubbing or kneading in a circular motion can relax muscles and bring warmth to sore areas. To let hands move smoothly over skin, use baby oil that has been warmed by setting the bottle in hot tap water (never heat the oil in a microwave). However, don't massage an already inflamed joint.

• **TENS.** In transcutaneous electrical nerve stimulation (TENS), the electrodes on a hand-held, battery-powered unit are taped to skin on or near the painful area. A low-level electrical stimulation is delivered for thirty minutes or up to two hours. The tingling sensation seems to trigger nerves to send out endorphins, changing your body's perception of pain. Though it sounds like science fiction, the technique is actually quite safe and easy to self-administer, but rent a unit and try it for a while before buying one for home use. You shouldn't undergo TENS if you have a pacemaker or if you're pregnant.

• **Biofeedback.** In this technique, your body's physical responses are electronically monitored; a series of beeps, a continuous tone or a computer-screen image follows the changes in your heart rate, skin temperature, even brain waves. You can then be trained to modify or slow down those patterns using visualization or other relaxation techniques. Once you've mastered control over your responses on the machine, you can use the same images to relax anywhere, anytime, to reduce your pain.

• **Hypnosis.** No longer just a magic-show trick, hypnosis has been shown to be an effective, medically sound approach to relaxation. When inducing a trance, you're alert yet are not aware of bodily sensations—similar to the feeling you have just before waking or falling asleep. Your doctor may be able to refer you to a psychiatrist or psychologist trained in this technique, who can also teach you how to put yourself into a hypnotic state when necessary.

Start a Pain Journal

Not every pain management strategy works for everyone. To develop a formula right for you, keep a pain journal. When pain strikes, write down the time of day it occurred, the activity you were engaged in and any other circumstances surrounding or preceding the flare. For instance, had you just finished a heavy meal, had an argument with a coworker, telephoned an ailing relative? Note how you reacted to the pain: Did you stop moving the joint, sit down, go to bed, take a drink? Record how the pain made you feel: angry, helpless, determined to overcome it? From these details, you may begin to notice a pattern that can help you change or avoid negative attitudes and behaviors.

As you begin to try out different treatments, note when your pain is relieved. Is it better after you take your medication, do your exercises, focus on other tasks? Do physical measures help, such as a massage when you ache, or cold packs for swelling? Can you rely on distractions—reading a book, singing along with the radio—to take your mind off persistent but mild discomfort? Are acute episodes, with their sharp but short-term pain, easier to deal with if you practice relaxation techniques such as deep breathing or yoga? Once you've amassed your arsenal of pain-stoppers, you'll be better equipped to control your arthritis.

CHAPTER 7

Using Medications

Most likely, your doctor will outline some type of drug therapy for you that will either help you through an arthritis flare or reduce the severity of your next one. The medications that have been developed can control many symptoms of arthritis and, in certain cases, can even halt its progression. However, you must understand that drug therapy is *not* a cure. It's just one part of a well-rounded treatment program that includes exercise and joint protection.

If you're not currently under a physician's care for arthritis, don't self-medicate. A friend who has joint pain may recommend aspirin or even offer to share her pills, but don't be swayed! Even if your symptoms are similar, your case of arthritis may be very different from your friend's and require a different dosage or drug. The effects of misused medicine—even the "harmless" ones available without a prescription—can be devastating, not only for your arthritis but for your overall health. Medication should only be taken under medical supervision.

Choosing the appropriate medicine requires your doctor's skill and experience along with your own input. It may take a few attempts to find the drug and the dose that give you the most benefit with the fewest side effects. Even if your regimen includes a medication that doesn't require a prescription, you'll need to schedule regular checkups with your doctor to be sure the drug is doing its job and is not causing complications.

Following are descriptions of the most common medications used in the treatment of arthritis—their purpose, possible adverse reactions, tips for avoiding such effects, and how the medications' actions may be influenced by other drugs or food. Drug therapy is often unpredictable: No two people will respond to the same medication in exactly the same way. Every medication has side effects, though you may experience only a few or none if you take them as directed. The potential problems mentioned here are the more common complaints, to help you tell whether something is wrong that needs to be reported to your doctor. However, these are just a few of many reactions; any changes in your health while taking these medications should be brought to your physician's attention immediately (for more precautions, see "Taking Responsibility" at the end of this chapter).

Salicylates

Salicylates, the class of drugs to which aspirin belongs, have been used to treat rheumatism for over a century, since they were found naturally in willow-tree bark and other plants. They can block the release of prostaglandins, the hormones produced when you have inflammation. Since salicylates reduce fever, relieve pain and suppress inflammation, they can counter the most common symptoms of all forms of arthritis—with fewer side effects and at less expense than other arthritis medications.

Aspirin

Inexpensive and effective, aspirin is the most common treatment for less severe discomfort. In small doses (two tablets every four to six hours), it's a pain reliever. In high doses (three or four tablets four to six times a day), it reduces inflammation.

Side effects: Irritates the gastrointestinal tract, causing mild to serious symptoms such as stomachache, nausea, heartburn and ulcers. Too-high doses can cause a ringing sensation in the ears (tinnitus) or temporary deafness, and dizziness. (The above reactions are not allergic; an allergic reaction usually seems to strike those with asthma or nasal polyps.) Aspirin also can affect the kidneys and liver, so may not be recommended for those who have impaired function of these organs. It thins the blood, and may result in excessive bleeding during surgery or dental work; on the other hand, this side effect may help prevent blood clots, and thus strokes or heart attacks.

Safety measures: To minimize stomach upset, take after meals or with milk or an antacid. Swallow with a full eight ounces of the milk or other liquid; don't lie down for fifteen to thirty minutes afterward. You may also ask your doctor whether you can take buffered, coated, timed-release or liquid aspirin, products that are easier on your stomach. If a tablet has a vinegary smell, discard; the medicine has begun to break down and won't be as effective. Other nonprescription drugs, such as cold remedies, and some prescription pain relievers also contain aspirin; if you use these products, check the ingredients list or ask your pharmacist to be sure you won't be overdosing with aspirin.

Interactions: Oral anticoagulants (blood-thinning drugs used to treat some heart conditions), oral corticosteroids and other NSAIDs (these anti-inflammatories are described below) and alcoholic beverages can increase gastric upset or bleeding. Aspirin should not be used with probenecid and sulfinpyrazone (gout medications; see below), and can interact with water pills, such as hydrochlorothiazide, given for hypertension or heart disease. Aspirin can increase the effect of methotrexate, an anticancer drug sometimes prescribed for severe arthritis (see "Cytotoxic Drugs," below).

Diflunisal, Choline Magnesium Trisalicylate, Salsalate

These salicylates cost more than aspirin and must be prescribed. However, they have the same but longer-lasting effect at half the dose, so are less likely to cause serious reaction and are usually better tolerated.

Side effects: Same as aspirin.

Safety measures: Take at the same time each day, on an empty stomach, if that can be tolerated.

Interactions: Same as aspirin.

Acetaminophen

Though not a salicylate, acetaminophen is often substituted by people who are allergic to or can't tolerate the side effects of aspirin. Be aware that this nonprescription drug acts only as a pain reliever, with no effect on inflammation, so it would benefit only the mild discomfort of early-stage osteoarthritis. Don't switch from aspirin to acetominophen without speaking to your doctor first.

Side effects: Safer than aspirin. Serious side effects are rare unless taken in extremely large amounts.

Safety measures: Should not be taken for more than ten days in a row (five for children) without consulting your physician.

Interactions: No serious interactions.

Nonsteroidal Anti-inflammatory Drugs (NSAIDs)

These medications decrease inflammation as corticosteroids do (see below) but without the severe side effects—hence the name. Second in frequency of use only to aspirin, NSAIDs also inhibit prostaglandin production. They are given for inflammatory diseases like rheumatoid arthritis, lupus and Sjögren's syndrome, and are also used to treat osteoarthritis.

NSAIDs have several advantages over aspirin: They can be taken less often (one to three times a day), so patients can keep to a more convenient dosing schedule; they cause less gastric distress or bleeding; and some are more effective for certain diseases. Disadvantages: They cost more, and all except ibuprofen must be prescribed.

Another drawback is that though there are many different NSAIDs, they don't all behave the same way and cannot predictably help each person with each type of arthritis. Therefore, it may take several tries with various NSAIDs before your doctor can find the one that provides the most relief for you.

If you're allergic to aspirin, you'll probably be allergic to the NSAIDs as well. All NSAIDs may interfere with the action of sulfa drugs (prescribed for infections), oral diabetes medications and phenytoin (used to treat seizures), and can increase lithium levels. Don't take any NSAID with warfarin (a blood-thinning drug prescribed for some heart conditions).

Ibuprofen, Fenoprofen, Fluriprofen, Ketoprofen, Naproxen

These drugs belong to the group called phenylopropionic acids.

Side effects: Upset stomach, nausea, heartburn; occasionally (especially with naproxen) fluid retention. In patients with lupus, ibuprofen can, though rarely, cause a form of meningitis with symptoms such as headache, fever and stiff neck. Fenoprofen is more likely, though still rarely, to affect the kidneys.

Safety measures: To counteract stomach irritation, take after meals or with an antacid.

Interactions: Don't take with aspirin or another NSAID.

Indomethacin, Sulindac, Tolmetin, Diclofenac, Etodolac

These related drugs—called acetic acid derivatives—are often prescribed to treat ankylosing spondylitis, gout and rheumatoid arthritis. Indomethacin and sulindac have also been shown to be effective for bursitis in the shoulder, and tolmetin improves some cases of juvenile arthritis. Diclofenac and etodolac are the most recently approved medications in this group.

Using Medications 95

Side effects: Gastrointestinal upset, fluid retention—though effects are less likely with sulindac and tolmetin. Indomethacin has been known to cause severe headache, light-headedness and confusion, ringing in the ears, and blurry or double vision. Diclofenac has been associated with liver damage.

Safety measures: Dose at the same time each day. Best if taken on an empty stomach, but if irritation results, take with food or an antacid. Reduce salt and sodium in your diet if bloating occurs. If you develop headaches, discontinue medicine and contact your doctor. If you're taking diclofenac, regular blood tests are needed to check effects on liver.

Interactions: Aspirin can interfere with absorption. Indomethacin can interfere with water pills.

Phenylbutazone

The first NSAID developed after aspirin, now this drug is generally used only for short-term, but effective, treatment of ankylosing spondylitis, gout, tendonitis or bursitis. In rare cases, it can decrease the number of blood cells the body can make, and so is often the NSAID of last resort.

Side effects: Stomach upset; rapid weight gain from the high level of fluid and salt retention—a particular problem for people with high blood pressure or heart disease. Can cause fatal blood conditions.

Safety measures: Take a half hour after meals or an antacid. You should undergo a blood test every few weeks. Do not take this medication for more than a week at a time.

Interactions: Do not take with aspirin or other arthritis drugs.

Meclofenamate

This medication may be prescribed for osteoarthritis, rheumatoid arthritis and other muscle or joint conditions.

Side effects: Can cause diarrhea, nausea or other stomach distress.

Safety measures: Take after food or with an antacid.

Interactions: Avoid alcohol, aspirin and other arthritis medications.

Piroxicam

Requiring only a once-a-day dose, this medicine can be effective against rheumatoid arthritis and osteoarthritis, gout and ankylosing spondylitis.

Side effects: In a few cases, stomachache. May make skin sensitive to the sun, causing a rash.

Safety measures: Take after meals or with an antacid.

Interactions: Avoid aspirin, and other NSAIDs, unless prescribed by your doctor.

Nabumetone

One of the newest NSAIDs to be approved in the United States, this drug is formulated to become active only after it reaches the liver, lessening its effects on the stomach.

Side effects: Minor gastrointestinal symptoms, such as upset stomach, indigestion, diarrhea. Less risk of serious gastric problems, such as ulcers or bleeding.

Safety measures: Can be taken on an empty stomach, but for long-term use take after meals or an antacid.

Interactions: Don't take with aspirin or other NSAIDs, unless directed by your doctor.

Corticosteroids

When rheumatoid arthritis patients were first given cortisone in 1949, their improvement was so dramatic that it was touted as a miracle drug—until its side effects came to light with long-term use. Now it's given chiefly to temporarily relieve rheumatoid arthritis flare-ups, or treat severe cases of lupus and other inflammatory diseases. It's not helpful for osteoarthritis.

Corticosteroids—the drug group that includes cortisone, as well as hydrocortisone (also called cortisol) and prednisone—are chemical derivatives of the human hormone produced by the adrenal glands. These medications not only suppress inflammation, they suppress, even stop, the hormone-making action of the adrenal glands; when they are to be discontinued, they must be withdrawn gradually to allow the glands to begin working on their own again. Doses may also have to be increased during times of stress, physical trauma or infection, when the glands would normally send out extra hormone.

Corticosteroids can be administered several ways. To minimize side effects, oral medications are more commonly given in one daily low-potency dose, or in slightly higher doses every other day. For some conditions, injections directly into the inflamed joint can produce the quickest results with the fewest side effects.

Side effects: Nervousness, insomnia; bloating, puffiness in the face from fluid retention; weight gain from increased appetite; acne, thinning of the skin; cataracts; high blood pressure. May reduce resistance to infection and slow healing, elevate blood sugar, draw calcium from bones and weaken muscles. In children, can slow growth. In rare cases, can cause psychosis.

Safety measures: To guard against weight gain, follow a

well-balanced diet, low in salt and calories. Be sure you also get enough calcium, found in dairy products, broccoli, kale and other greens; talk to your doctor before taking a calcium supplement. Injections can eventually damage bones, so most medical experts recommend no more than three shots in one site, with doses no less than four weeks apart. If you have diabetes, osteoporosis, peptic ulcer, high blood pressure, heart disease or a psychiatric disorder, you are not an ideal candidate for corticosteroids.

Interactions: If you're taking medications for diabetes, high blood pressure or glaucoma, steroids can make these conditions more difficult to control. Avoid alcoholic beverages. Aspirin and other arthritis drugs should be used only if also prescribed by your physician. The corticosteroid *prednisone* cannot be as readily absorbed if taken with an antacid.

Disease-Modifying Antirheumatic Drugs (DMARDs)

As potent as the corticosteroids, these medications are usually reserved for more severe cases that don't respond to the salicylates or NSAIDs. Recently they have begun to be used also in earlier stages of diseases where many joints are involved, such as rheumatoid arthritis, because DMARDs have been shown to slow down, and even reverse, joint destruction. How this is accomplished is not yet known.

These drugs are also known as slow-acting antirheumatic drugs because improvements usually are not noticeable until after months of treatment. However, results last long after a DMARD is stopped. The serious side effects of DMARDs require that doctors be cautious in administering them, and they should be prescribed only by a rheumatologist or other physician experienced in their use.

Gold Salts

These compounds are most often used for rheumatoid arthritis, as well as juvenile and psoriatic arthritis. They may be injected into a muscle or taken by mouth.

Side effects: Cold sweats, flushing, dizziness, fainting, nausea. May leave a metallic taste in your mouth. Can trigger mouth sores and skin rash when injected, or diarrhea when taken orally. In some cases, kidneys can become damaged, releasing protein into the urine; bone marrow may stop producing certain blood cells, which can result in an increased risk of infection or uncontrollable bleeding.

Safety measures: Because of the chance of fainting, gold injections should be given while you're lying down; remain in that position for about fifteen minutes afterward. Your condition should be carefully monitored with regular blood and urine tests.

Penicillamine

A very distant relative of penicillin (and without its infection-fighting power), this DMARD is used for juvenile and adult rheumatoid arthritis. Further study is needed to prove its helpfulness in treating scleroderma.

Side effects: Fever, skin rash, mouth sores, loss of taste and appetite, nausea. Can also affect blood cell production and kidneys. Very rarely, may trigger an unusual medical condition, such as myasthenia gravis or Goodpasture's syndrome.

Safety measures: Take one hour before or two hours after meals, or at least an hour before other food, milk or medicines, as they can interfere with absorption. Regular blood and urine tests are needed to monitor this drug's effects.

Interactions: If you're allergic to penicillin, you're not at risk of an allergic reaction to penicillamine.

Antimalarial Drugs

For reasons still unclear, chloroquine and hydroxychloroquine not only work for malaria; these drugs can also control the symptoms of lupus, rheumatoid arthritis and Sjögren's syndrome. They are slightly less effective than gold or penicillamine treatments, but have fewer side effects and can be continued for many years.

Side effects: Heartburn, nausea, vomiting, skin rash or discoloration occasionally may occur. In high doses for long periods, vision problems can occur such as blurring, difficulty in focusing or seeing to read, or blindness, but these conditions are usually reversible if caught early.

Safety measures: Take at the same time each day, on an empty stomach if possible, or with milk or after food to prevent gastric problems. Eyes should be examined by an ophthalmologist every six months. Wear sunglasses outdoors, when possible, as sunlight seems to add to the risk of vision problems.

Sulfasalazine

This medication is chemically related to both aspirin and sulfa antibiotics. Used to treat inflammatory bowel diseases such as colitis, it also has been found to reduce inflammation in the spondyloarthropathies.

Side effects: Gastrointestinal problems such as nausea, stomach upset and diarrhea, but not ulcers. Has been associated with anemia in some people.

Safety measures: Coated preparations are better tolerated. Be patient, as this medication takes several weeks to work. If you're allergic to other sulfa drugs, you will be allergic to sulfasalazine.

Cytotoxic Drugs

These powerful medicines are usually used to fight cancer or to prevent the body from rejecting an organ transplant: They're poisonous to certain cells and suppress the immune system. As strong immunosuppressants, they also hold back the inflammation process, which is why they found their way into arthritis treatment. Most often, cytotoxic drugs are prescribed for severe rheumatoid arthritis, lupus and other connective tissue diseases when the benefits clearly outweigh the risks—for instance, when complications develop that might cause irreparable organ damage or death. These medications are not appropriate for osteoarthritis.

Unfortunately, the cytotoxics also kill off some beneficial cells, such as those in the bone marrow. By suppressing the immune system, they keep the body from fighting other infections that may be life-threatening. Dosages are kept low to reduce these risks.

Methotrexate

This medication is more commonly given than the other cytotoxics, as it works more quickly and its side effects are easier to tolerate for most people. Given in pill form or by injection, it's used to treat rheumatoid arthritis, juvenile rheumatoid arthritis, psoriatic arthritis and Reiter's syndrome.

Side effects: Mouth sores, nausea, cramps, vomiting, diarrhea, hair loss. Reduces blood cell production, which can result in frequent infections or bleeding disorders. In some cases, can impair liver function.

Safety measures: Take at the same time for each once-a-week dose, on an empty stomach if possible. Have regular blood tests. Drinking extra fluids can help the kidneys pass the drug more quickly and safely. You should not take this drug if you have a history of liver disease.

Interactions: Aspirin and the infection medications tetracycline, chloramphenicol and sulfonamides can increase the severity of side effects. Limit alcoholic beverages, as they can also irritate the liver.

Azathioprine

This cytotoxic drug is prescribed for rheumatoid arthritis and other inflammatory conditions, in particular lupus and polymyositis.

Side effects: Fatigue, fever, chills, stomach upset, loss of appetite. May increase risk of infection or liver damage. After long use, may raise risk of cancer.

Safety measures: For best results, take on an empty stomach if possible. Monthly blood tests are needed.

Interactions: Not to be taken with allopurinol (a gout medication; see below), which can dangerously increase the release of azathioprine into the blood.

Cyclophosphamide

As the strongest of the cytotoxic drugs, this also has the most serious side effects. Sometimes taken for RA, it is also used to treat kidney-affected lupus and inflammations of the blood vessels, given intravenously or orally. It may be prescribed in smaller doses in combination with corticosteroids.

Side effects: Temporary hair loss, nausea, vomiting, loss of appetite. This drug can also affect fertility; sometimes this effect is permanent. At high doses or over long periods, bloody or painful urination can occur. Increases risk of infection, kidney damage, leukemia and bladder cancer.

Safety measures: To minimize irritation of the bladder and kidneys, drink eight extra eight-ounce cups of water daily, and empty your bladder frequently. Cyclophosphamide works best if taken in the morning so that the drug does not stay in the bladder overnight. Schedule frequent blood tests.

Cyclosporine

This is another very powerful cytotoxic drug that suppresses the immune system. Recent experiments have found it helpful in treating some cases of rheumatoid arthritis and lupus. It has many serious side effects and so must be prescribed with caution.

Gout Medications

In most cases, gout can be easily managed through diet (see Chapter 9) and the prescription medications that follow.

Colchicine

Other NSAIDs may also be prescribed, but colchicine is most often given to block inflammation, for quick relief of a gout attack. In some cases, your doctor may prescribe smaller doses to be taken every day to prevent flares, along with the other gout medications below. This ancient drug, still made from the saffron plant, can be injected or taken in pill form.

Side effects: Cramps, nausea or vomiting, severe diarrhea, particularly with the higher oral doses. Redness, swelling or pain at injection site.

Safety measures: Begin taking immediately at the first sign of an attack; stop treatment once the flare subsides or if side effects begin. Eat a well-balanced diet and drink plenty of water to replace nutrients and fluids lost through diarrhea.

Interaction: Avoid alcoholic beverages.

Uricosuric Agents

For chronic gout, probenecid or sulfinpyrazone may be prescribed to increase the elimination of uric acid through the urine. They are usually begun *between* gout attacks, or else they can worsen a flare. They also prevent the formation of tophi, the bumpy deposits of uric acid crystals under the skin.

Side effects: Headache, loss of appetite, nausea or mild vomiting, cramps, skin rash, bloody or painful urination. Can trigger a gout attack. Can increase kidney stones.

Safety measures: Results may not be obvious for a few months, so be patient. Drink ten to twelve eight-ounce glasses of water each day, to help move uric acid out of your body and prevent kidney stones.

Interactions: Avoid aspirin and alcoholic beverages, which block the drugs' action. Probenecid increases the effects of the antibiotic penicillin and the blood-thinning drug heparin.

Allopurinol

This medication slows the production of uric acid by blocking the enzyme that creates the acid. Most commonly prescribed for those with very high uric acid levels in the blood, it can also dissolve tophi.

Side effects: Allergic reaction, such as skin rash, hives or itching, sometimes with fever; hair loss, diarrhea, drowsiness or impaired alertness, blood abnormalities. In rare cases, kidney stones may form.

Safety measures: Works after a few months. Drink ten to twelve eight-ounce glasses of water daily to reduce the chance of kidney stones. Blood should be regularly tested to check uric acid levels.

Interactions: Alcohol can hamper the drug's effectiveness. Large doses of vitamin C may increase the risk of kidney stones. Thiazide diuretics (for high blood pressure) can raise the risk of side effects. Don't take with azathioprine.

Antidepressants

In some cases of arthritis, a tricyclic antidepressant such as doxepin may be prescribed for its effects as a pain reliever or to help with sleep. Doses are small and are not meant to lift mental depression, though they may have some effect on your mood.

Side effects: Dizziness, drowsiness, dry mouth, headache, blurred vision, constipation, fainting, rapid heartbeat.

Safety measures: Best if taken before bedtime. If medication makes you drowsy, do not drive, use machinery or perform any activity that can be dangerous if alertness is impaired.

Interactions: If you're on a tricyclic antidepressant, you should not also take an MAO inhibitor, also prescribed for depression. Alcoholic beverages and antihistamines (in allergy or cold remedies) can increase drowsiness.

Muscle Relaxants

In rheumatoid arthritis, drugs such as cyclobenzaprine or carisoprodol may be given to reduce the pressure of muscle spasms near affected joints. They have no direct effect on joint pain or inflammation.

Side effects: Blurred vision, light-headedness, drowsiness, depression.

Safety measures: While under the influence of such medications, don't drive, use machinery or perform any activity that can be dangerous if your vision or alertness is impaired.

Interactions: If you're on a muscle relaxant, you should not also take an MAO inhibitor (prescribed for depression). Alcoholic beverages and antihistamines (in allergy or cold remedies) can increase drowsiness.

Narcotics

Narcotics like codeine may be prescribed as a pain reliever, but are not recommended because they can be addictive, especially when taken long-term for a chronic illness like arthritis. Sometimes codeine is added to aspirin to boost its effectiveness as a painkiller; it does not help with inflammation.

Side effects: Drowsiness, loss of alertness, dizziness, headache, nausea, dry mouth, loss of appetite, depression, constipation. Can be habit-forming.

Safety measures: While under the influence of such medications, don't drive, use machinery or perform any activity that requires you to be alert.

Interactions: MAO inhibitors (antidepressants), alcoholic beverages, cough medicines, and cold and allergy remedies containing antihistamines can increase the sedative effect.

Anesthetics

Sometimes an anesthetic such as lidocaine or procaine may be mixed with an injected corticosteroid—to give immediate pain relief in a joint such as the shoulder before the arthritis drug can take effect.

Side effects: In a few cases, allergic reaction, such as skin rash or hives.

Safety measures: Be careful to avoid injuring the numbed area before the anesthetic wears off.

Taking Responsibility

Once your doctor writes you a prescription, it will be up to you to be sure you know how to take the medication correctly and to comply with any directions for its use. Doctors don't always take the time to go over all you need to know, so you may have to gather some information yourself. (To keep track of this data, make copies of the Medication Fact Sheet that follows, and fill one out for each of your arthritis remedies; actually it's a good idea to have these facts on hand for any drug you take regularly, even over-the-counter pharmaceuticals.) Your pharmacist can also answer questions about a drug that you may have forgotten to ask in the doctor's office. These guidelines will help you medicate safely and wisely.

• Know the drug's name. If it's not readable on the prescription form, have the doctor or nurse print it legibly. Be sure you have both the brand name (given by the manufacturer) and the generic (chemical) name; for instance, Motrin is a brand of the generic drug ibuprofen. In the drug descriptions in this chapter, only generics have been given; there may be several brand names for a drug and different doctors may prescribe different products or the generic. That's why it's best to know both names.

• Know whether your pharmacist has substituted a generic drug for a brand name. Depending on state law, a pharmacist may be able to make the change to a generic without consulting your physician. Most generics are chemically identical to the brand names and are less expensive, but some are not and may not be as effective for you. Check with your doctor.

• Educate yourself. Find out everything you can about the medication you're taking: its purpose; side effects; possible interactions with other drugs, vitamins or food; when is the best time to take it; how long before it takes effect, etc. Get the answers from your doctor or pharmacist, or check your public library for reference books such as *About Your Medicines* or *USP DI Volume II: Advice for the Patient* (both published by the U.S. Pharmacopeial Convention), or *Physicians' Desk Reference* (Medical Economics Co.). If you can read the fine print, you can also glean some of this information from the package insert included by the drug manufacturer, available from your doctor or pharmacist.

• Follow directions exactly. Take only the dosage recommended, at the time of day suggested, and with or without food as advised. If your doctor wasn't specific, ask questions. If the label instructions aren't clear to you, your pharmacist can help you interpret them. For instance, if the label reads, "Take two tablets four times a day," does that mean during your waking hours only, or should you take the pills every six hours, getting up in the night for your last dose?

• Never skimp on a medicine to save money, or increase your dosage, assuming that more is better. These are dangerous practices that can worsen your arthritis and threaten your health.

• Stay on schedule. If you miss a dose or two, don't just forget about it or double up on your next dose. Contact your doctor or pharmacist to find out how to get back on track.

• Report your reactions. If the medication makes you sick to your stomach or dizzy, if symptoms don't improve or you feel worse than before, tell your doctor. Some side effects are expected and require no attention; others could be signs of trouble. Your physician knows the difference.

• Tell your doctor about your other medications. If you're seeing several doctors for different conditions, be sure that each is aware of the various prescriptions you may already be taking. Bring a list of the names and dosages, or bring the containers themselves to your physician. This should include any nonprescription drugs you use regularly, such as aspirin, allergy medicines and menstrual pain relievers. They, too, can interfere with the action of your medicines or create a harmful interaction.

• If your doctor prescribes a different arthritis medication, stop taking your previous arthritis remedy unless instructed otherwise. Combining drugs won't make you feel better and will probably do more harm.

• Inform your arthritis doctor immediately if you are pregnant, or plan on becoming pregnant, or are breastfeeding. Any medication, including aspirin, can affect a developing fetus or be passed into breast milk. Your physician may have to change your dosage or discontinue your medication.

• It bears repeating: Never take a friend's or relative's medication, and never give someone else yours.

Medication Fact Sheet

Generic name: _____

Brand name: _____

Prescription number: _____

Dosage amount: _____

When to take: _____

_____

How to take (with food/water/other liquids/on empty stomach): _____

_____

When drug will take effect: _____

When to stop taking: _____

How to make up for a missed dose: _____

_____

Expected side effects: _____

_____

How to treat side effects: _____

_____

Potentially harmful side effects: _____

_____

_____

Effect on nutrients (vitamins/minerals): _____

_____

Other drugs, prescription and nonprescription, to avoid: _____

_____

_____

Foods and beverages to avoid: _____

_____

Other instructions or precautions: _____

_____

_____

CHAPTER 8

Opting for Surgery

For most people with arthritis, a well-balanced program of exercise, rest, joint protection and drug therapy can help them manage their disease throughout their lives. However, if your condition is severe or cannot be controlled, surgery may be the only way to repair an ailing joint and alleviate symptoms.

The past two decades have brought incredible advances in arthritis surgery. Hundreds of thousands of total joint replacement operations are performed every year in the United States. This and other surgical procedures offer tremendous relief from pain, greater mobility and an overall better quality of life. Still, surgery is not without risk and so is often considered a treatment of last resort.

Generally, surgical treatment may be suggested for one or a combination of the following reasons:

• **Your pain fails to respond to other therapies.** This may be the most compelling reason for surgery, as severe, persistent pain can be disabling, interfering with the simplest activities. Usually in these cases, a joint, cartilage, bone or connective tissue such as a tendon has been extensively damaged—a condition that can't be corrected by medication or physical therapy. With surgery, most people can expect freedom from pain.

• **A joint's range of motion is very limited.** When you can't move your arms to wash yourself or swing out your leg to walk, for example, your shoulder or hip has lost enough of its function that you become disabled. Several surgical techniques can make movement easier. Be aware, though, that the degree of mobility that can be restored by the surgery must be carefully calculated beforehand, but is still unpredictable. It's unlikely that you'll regain 100 percent flexibility in the joint, but certainly most cases show vast improvement.

• **Damage is likely to progress.** If your doctor determines that your condition is worsening, he or she may recommend certain procedures, such as a synovectomy (described below), to prevent further damage to joints. In some circumstances, you may be advised to undergo an operation at an earlier stage of arthritis, before your condition has made you too weak to withstand the physical stress of surgery.

• **The joint is deformed.** When a joint's structure changes—cartilage is worn away or tendons weakened by inflammation, for instance—the bones may shift out of alignment; the result may be crippling. Some deformities, such as fingers misshapen by rheumatoid arthritis, may not be painful or interfere much with the joint's function, and so might not be worth the discomfort, inconvenience and cost of surgery to improve their appearance. However, if you feel embarrassed by the deformity, the boost to your self-esteem should be weighed in the balance.

Before your doctor recommends surgical treatment, he or she must take into account your age, overall health and attitude, including your willness to comply with instructions before and after an operation. But it will be you who makes the final decision to have surgery.

Except when a tendon has torn, or a bone is infected or pressing on nerves, surgery for arthritis is rarely an emergency. You should take whatever time you need to decide whether you want to undergo a surgical procedure. Know exactly how the operation will help you and how much return of function or relief from pain you can expect. Surgery is more often successful for the larger joints or when only one joint is involved. In addition, any surgery carries risks of other complications regardless of its effect on your arthritis. Blood clots that can block blood flow to the heart, severe blood loss or an adverse reaction to a blood transfusion are potential dangers. Though postoperative infections occur much less frequently than in the past, an infection from bacteria entering the surgical site is not unusual and can be life-threatening to a vulnerable patient. Other points to consider are discussed in "Your Role in Surgery," at the end of this chapter.

Descriptions of the most common surgical procedures follow, including in what circumstances and for which joints each might be appropriate.

Arthroplasty

In some cases, a joint may have to be surgically recon-
structed to restore stability or motion, or to eliminate
pain. This can be done several ways.

Total Joint Replacement

Now the best known and most important of the arthritis
surgeries, this technique involves substituting a man-
made joint for your damaged joint. In hip replacement, for
instance, a durable plastic, such as polyethylene, takes the
place of cartilage in the joint socket, while a metal ball on
a shaft takes the place of the rounded bone end of the other
half of the joint. These components are embedded into the
bone on either side and secured with a supercement. (A
new cementless technique to stabilize a replacement joint
also shows promise and is discussed below.)

In osteoarthritis and rheumatoid arthritis, the total replacement is most commonly and successfully done for the
hip joint, afterward allowing easier, pain-free sitting,
standing and walking. The knee is a more complicated
joint, and so the gains in movement after surgery may not
be as dramatic as the relief from pain; the fitting and
alignment of the different components must be precise, so
knee replacement should be performed by a surgeon well
skilled in this operation. Shoulder replacements bring
moderate improvement in function, with no pain. For
ankle replacements, the results have been mixed, and seem
to be best if the joint is not already out of alignment.
Because elbow replacements tend to become dislocated,
they're usually reserved for those who have severe RA or
are over age seventy and have osteoarthritis. The small

joints of the fingers can also be replaced, with hinge-like implants that greatly improve appearance; in most cases, the fingers are also much more flexible but may not be any stronger than before. Replacement of a wrist may be considered if tendons have not been damaged and the joint will not be put under too much stress.

While artificial joints are designed to withstand decades of pressure, they *can* wear out, and they, too, may have to be replaced eventually. In the past, surgeons were hesitant to put a hip joint replacement in anyone under forty-five because the joint was likely to loosen after years of weight bearing. However, a new cementless technique has been developed that may prove to be more reliable: The artificial joint is created with "pores," which allows new bone to grow into these spaces to hold the joint in place.

Partial Joint Replacement

In this procedure, as the name implies, only part of the joint is rebuilt. Though once performed more commonly on the hip, this procedure proved less beneficial and long-lasting than a total replacement. Today, a knee affected by osteoarthritis is more likely to be only partially replaced if only half of the joint is damaged.

Resurfacing

In this procedure, usually performed on the hip, the ball end of the damaged joint is smoothed down and covered with a metal cap. The socket is enlarged and fitted with a plastic insert that is bigger and thinner than those used in total joint replacement.

This procedure has two advantages: Bone is preserved,

so weight is distributed more naturally; and the components won't loosen, as is possible in total joint replacement. However, it also has its drawbacks: This operation could make later joint replacement more difficult and increase the chance of complications; there's no easy way to see what is happening to the bone under the metal cap, though this may be of more concern in rheumatoid arthritis. Still, this may be the better route for younger patients, to avoid a total joint replacement.

Resection

When a deformed bone gets in the way of easy movement, it may be cut out, partially or totally, without being replaced. This procedure is usually performed on bones that are not necessary for support or mobility. A common resectioning involves the big toe knuckle, or the bone on the inside of the wrist. A pseudoarthrosis—false joint—develops between the two bone ends. Pain disappears and often flexibility improves.

Arthrodesis

In some cases, joint bones are surgically encouraged to fuse, to remain rigid forever. The bone ends are cut, and are held in place while they grow together. This makes them stronger, more stable and better able to support your weight, free from pain.

The procedure is recommended for bones that are deformed but not eligible for reconstructive surgery. Included are the spine, ankle, wrist and some other bones of the foot and hand, where a loss of flexibility would be barely disabling. Performed on an elbow, hip or knee, though, arthrodesis would take away much of the joint's ability to function and is rarely done except as a last resort. However, a younger person who has this operation would still be able to have a total joint replacement later in life.

Arthroscopy

As you learned in Chapter 3, an arthroscope is a pencil-sized telescope that can be inserted to examine the inside of a joint, often to assess the damage there and determine a diagnosis. This instrument can also be used in surgery: Tiny "microtools" can be slipped through a separate hole in the arthroscope to operate on structures within the joint. The powerful scope can also be fitted with a lens that gives the surgeon an enlarged view of the operation's progress on a video screen. Because this procedure requires only a small incision, it offers tremendous advantages: minimal scarring, lower risk of infection, less pain, a shorter hospital stay and quicker recovery.

Arthroscopy is most often performed on the knee, to remove bits of debris like bone or cartilage that may be irritating the synovium and worsening inflammation. It is also used to scrape away bone spurs, resurface a joint, remove the joint lining (synovectomy; see below), or repair ligaments.

Synovectomy

As explained in Chapter 2, the synovium or pannus (overgrown synovium) releases chemicals during inflammation that can erode connective tissues. One way to stop that from continuing is to remove the synovium. This procedure shows even better results in the earlier stages of rheumatoid arthritis before significant cartilage damage has occurred (for example, when inflammation has persisted for six months without relief from other therapies). Synovectomy can be especially beneficial for knees, wrists and knuckles.

However, after synovectomy, the joint may become stiff. In addition, the membrane often grows back, renewing pain and inflammation, though sometimes not as severely. The procedure may best be considered when only one joint cannot be controlled or when a toxic drug is the only alternative.

Synovium grows, too, along the tendons or bursae; if inflamed, it can erode these tissues and so may also be removed, in a procedure called tenosynovectomy. A chronically, painfully inflamed bursa can also be taken out (bursectomy), though this condition poses no threat of further damage to joints.

Osteotomy

When one area of a joint has been worn down by osteoarthritis, the solution may be to manually move it. Bone is cut and the joint is realigned, so that the less worn spot will now bear the weight—without pain. The bone must stay in this exact position for the six-to-eight-week healing process; rehabilitation may take another three to four months.

This operation is performed most often on the hip and knee, in patients under age sixty-five. The results last for about ten years.

Surgery on Tendons and Nerves

Sometimes the changes brought on by arthritis can cause pain in the tissues that surround the joint. A tendon, which connects the joint and helps it move, may tear, become inflamed or shift out of position. It can be repaired, reattached for better alignment or moved out of harm's way. Nerves, too, can become trapped by an arthritic joint, as by the wrist in carpal tunnel syndrome, and have to be released surgically.

Your Role in Surgery

Before and after an operation, you may have to take steps and make choices that will affect its success. You should be aware of these areas of concern even before giving your consent to surgery, as some may figure in your decision.

• Undergo a thorough physical examination to determine whether you are an ideal candidate for surgery. If you have heart or lung disease, for instance, you may not be fit for an operation. Some other conditions, such as dental cavities or a yeast infection, may have to be cleared up before you can undergo surgery; they can raise your risk of postoperative infection.

• Choose a surgeon with extensive experience in your procedure. Your regular physician will not be performing your surgery but instead will recommend an orthopedic surgeon or other specialist, depending on which procedure has been recommended. Before you decide on a surgeon, ask to speak to other patients who have had the same operation.

• Seek out a second, even a third, opinion. Often your insurance carrier will insist upon, and pay for, a second evaluation. It's to your benefit to consult with another surgeon to see whether the procedure recommended is best for your condition or whether surgery is needed at all. However, don't keep searching around until you find someone who says what you want to hear. If two doctors don't agree, a third should clinch it, or your rheumatologist can help you sort out your options.

• Decide on a hospital where procedures like yours are performed frequently. Such a facility will be better able to look after your needs while you're in its care.

• Educate yourself about the procedure, its benefits and complications. The outcome of some procedures can't be guaranteed, and you should be prepared for any eventuality. Know how long the surgery and recovery will take, whether additional surgery will be needed later and what type of follow-up therapy will be required.

• Plan how you will manage your recovery period. For months after your surgery, you may not be able to walk, drive a car or go to work. You may need special equipment, or have to rearrange your living areas so that you don't have to climb stairs to get to bed or maneuver crutches around furniture. Pressures may mount physically, financially and psychologically. Will you be able to handle them? Consider these obstacles before scheduling surgery and make appropriate arrangements before you enter the hospital.

• Educate your family and discuss with them what role they'll play in your recovery. Any surgery requires certain restrictions afterward, and family members will have to take up the slack. They may need to administer your medication or assist you in physical therapy. If this might be too much of a burden, it may be wise to arrange for outside help.

• Get healthy. Eat nutritiously, get plenty of rest and do your exercises—a fit body handles surgery much better and recovers much more quickly. Lose weight if necessary, as obesity complicates surgery and rehabilitation. Many surgeons won't perform a joint replacement if you're overweight, since the artificial joint is bound to fail under the extra burden.

• Be sure you know whether you should discontinue your arthritis medications before surgery. Some of these drugs, such as aspirin, prevent clotting, which can cause excessive bleeding during an operation and delay healing afterward. Others, like the corticosteroids and cytotoxic drugs, increase the risk of developing an infection, because they kill off infection-fighting white blood cells.

• Be willing to follow all instructions for your well-being after the operation. You'll probably have to stick to a strict regimen of rest, medication and physical therapy in the months after surgery. If you feel that you may not be able to adhere to such a program, you should reconsider having an operation, as it may do you little good.

In many cases, a patient's failure to participate in proper rehabilitation leaves the joint no more functional—or even worse off—than before, even though the surgery was successful.

• Maintain a positive attitude. Full recovery and rehabilitation after major surgery can take many months. Patients with rheumatoid arthritis who have major surgery spend about fourteen days in the hospital, and undergo two to six or more procedures during their lifetime. Under these circumstances, you may well become discouraged and wonder whether the end justified the means. Your cooperation and participation are essential in your treatment, and your recovery will be quicker and much more successful if you believe in yourself.

CHAPTER 9

The Role of Diet

Perhaps the most controversial area of arthritis treatment, at least among patients, is the effect of certain foods on their condition. Many people swear that tomatoes or dairy products trigger their flares. Others are sure that a vitamin deficiency must be at the root of their symptoms. Unfortunately, scientific studies have turned up little to support either of these claims, at least not enough to offer hope to most arthritis sufferers.

That's not to say that the foods you eat regularly don't have some influence on arthritis. For anyone, good nutrition is essential to good health; for someone already weakened by arthritis, eating properly is especially important, to prevent the condition from deteriorating further. Malnutrition can aggravate symptoms and increase the risk of serious complications. However, diet does not cause arthritis and no one food or combination of foods or particular vitamin will cure it.

Diet and Gout

Only gout has a clear-cut connection to diet. Those who suffer from this type of arthritis have a high blood level of uric acid—the waste product of purines, the compounds found in meats, seafood, beans and some vegetables. Eating high-purine foods can increase a gout patient's uric acid level by 20 to 30 percent. While gout medications are often the most effective way to lower uric acid levels (see Chapter 7), a change in diet alone may help. Even if you're on drug therapy, your doctor may advise you to limit foods that contain purines (see chart below). The best diet for those with gout appears to be one low in calories and fat, with restricted purines (eliminating them entirely is usually not necessary) and moderate intake of protein in general (less than three ounces a day). Often, overindulgence in rich foods (high in fats or purines) or alcoholic beverages (heavy wines or champagnes, in particular) can bring on a gout attack.

Obesity and Arthritis

A different aspect of diet that also has a direct effect on arthritis is obesity. When you take in more calories than your body uses up through everyday activity and exercise, the excess is stored as fat. If you don't reduce your eating or increase your exercise, pounds will continue to accumulate. In medical terms, an obese person weighs more than 20 percent over his or her ideal weight.

While obesity can be a consequence of arthritis for those who limit their activity because of pain or who use food to comfort themselves, it may also be a factor in the develop-

Purine Content of Foods
Amounts are given in milligrams per 100 grams of food
(equal to a 3½-ounce portion).

1. Very High in Purines (150–1,000 mg)		2. High in Purines (75–150 mg)	
Yeast	570–990	Anchovies	Partridge
Herring roe	484	Bacon	Pheasant
Sweetbreads	426	Codfish	Pigeon
Meat extracts	236–356	Goose	Salmon
Sardines	234	Grouse	Scallops
Heart, sheep	174	Haddock	Trout
Herring	172	Kidneys	Turkey
Smelts	168	Liver	Veal
Mussels	154	Mackerel	Venison

3. Moderately High in Purines (up to 75 mg)		4. Little or No Purines	
Asparagus	Lobster	Beverages	Pies (except
Bass	Mushrooms	(coffee,	mincemeat)*
Beef	Navy beans	cocoa,	Sugar*
Bouillon	Oysters	fruit juices,	Sweets*
Brains	Peas	soft drinks,	Vegetable or
Chicken	Pork	tea)	cream
Crab		Breads,	soups
Duck		crackers	not made
		Butter*	with List 3

3. Moderately High in Purines (up to 75 mg)

4. Little or No Purines

3. Moderately High in Purines (up to 75 mg)		4. Little or No Purines	
Eel	Rabbit	Caviar	vegetables
Halibut	Roe	Cereals and	or meat
Ham	Shrimp	cereal products	stock
Kidney beans	Spinach	(pasta, hominy	Vegetables
Lentils	Tongue	arrowroot)	not in
Lima beans	Tripe	Cheeses, all kinds*	List 3
Liverwurst		Eggs	
		Fats, all kinds*	
		Fruit, all kinds	
		Milk	
		Nuts, nut butters	

*High in fats, or high in calories that offer little nutritional value. Limit consumption.

Adapted from: Hench, P. S.: In Cecil, R. L., and Loeb, R. F. (eds.): *Textbook of Medicine*, 9th ed. From Bridges, M. A.: *Food and Beverage Analyses*, 3rd ed. Philadelphia, Lea & Febiger, 1950, pp. 188–92; and Dirr, K., and Decker, P.: *Biochem. Z.* 316:239, 1944.

ment of certain rheumatic diseases. For instance, those who are overweight are at greater risk of gout; the heavier you are, the more likely it is that you'll develop it. About 40 percent of those with gout are 10 percent over normal weight.

In addition, osteoarthritis occurs twice as often among people who are obese than among those of normal weight. Certainly extra pounds can stress weight-bearing joints such as hips and knees, worsening symptoms and speeding up damage to cartilage. But for some reason, the association of obesity with osteoarthritis seems to hold for non-weight-bearing joints as well.

Recipe for Good Health

If you have arthritis, you should be concerned about keeping to a healthy diet. Your body needs many nutrients—the twelve essential vitamins as well as minerals and trace elements—to maintain and repair itself. When the body is not properly nourished, the immune system can falter—already a problem for those who have autoimmune disorders like rheumatoid arthritis and lupus. This further worsens inflammation and slows healing. Well-balanced meals provide the energy that fights off fatigue, the enemy of those who suffer chronic pain. The right food choices can prevent some consequences of inactivity (such as heart disease, hypertension, overweight and constipation) and offset the side effects of some arthritis drugs (water retention, calcium loss).

What is a healthy diet? The U.S. Department of Health and Human Services and the Department of Agriculture (USDA) spelled it out in their 1990 "Dietary Guidelines for Americans." These recommendations are beneficial not only for general well-being, but for arthritis as well.

• **Eat a variety of foods.** Chronic illness and the medications used to treat them can rob you of certain vitamins and minerals (see "Nutritional Supplements" below). To ensure that you get all the nutrients your body requires, you must vary your menu. Vitamin or mineral supplements should not be substitutes for well-balanced eating; the natural composition and combinations of nutrients from food are more effectively and efficiently handled by the body. The best regimen includes different green leafy vegetables; yellow and orange vegetables (carrots, sweet potatoes); fruits high in vitamin C (strawberries and melon, and oranges, grapefruit and other citrus); whole grains and breads; lean meats, poultry and seafood; low-fat milk, yogurt, cheese and other dairy products.

• **Maintain a desirable weight.** As explained above, gout and osteoarthritis are linked to obesity. But for other forms of arthritis, *underweight* may be a problem. Chronic pain may leave you with little appetite. Limited movement may prevent you from regularly shopping for or preparing well-balanced meals. If your upper-body joints are affected, you may have difficulty even lifting food to your mouth or chewing. Under these circumstances, you may not only be 10 percent under normal weight, you may also be suffering from malnutrition.

Your "desirable" weight is not how much you would like to weigh, but what is appropriate for your height, sex and build. Your doctor can offer you guidelines based on current height-weight charts. Or you can quickly estimate your ideal weight this way: If you're an adult female, allow 100 pounds for your first 5 feet of height, then add 5 pounds for each inch over that (or subtract 5 for each inch under); if you're an adult male, figure 110 pounds for the first 5 feet. Add 10 percent of the total to that figure if you're large-boned, or subtract 10 percent for a small frame. For example: The ideal weight for a small-boned 5-foot, 4-inch woman would be 108 pounds; a 5-foot, 10-inch man with a large frame should weigh 176.

If you do need to lose or gain pounds, do so under your doctor's guidance. You need to be sure that your diet gives you enough nutrients and that your weight change will be gradual. Sudden fluctuations in weight can affect your condition. In gout, for instance, attacks can be triggered by crash dieting or fasting, which forces the body to burn proteins for energy, creating higher levels of uric acid in the blood.

• **Avoid too much fat, saturated fat and cholesterol.** Because dietary fats, or lipids, are involved in the formation of the chemicals that affect inflammation, immunity and collagen production, scientists believe these substances may play a role in arthritis treatment. Still, more research needs to be done in this area. However, in gout, high-fat foods are known to interfere with the elimination of uric acid from the kidneys, and should be avoided.

As important for arthritis sufferers, though, is cutting down on fats to lower the risk of heart disease. If your condition keeps you from getting enough aerobic exercise (as discussed in Chapter 5), you also increase your chances of cardiovascular problems. Heart disease is the number-one cause of death among gout patients. Several types of arthritis—including rheumatoid arthritis and lupus—also affect the cardiovascular system. Saturated fats in the diet raise the amount of cholesterol in the body; this fat-like substance deposits on blood vessel walls, clogging arteries and further straining the heart. These cholesterol-boosting fats come from animal products (meat, butter, cheese, milk, lard, solid shortening) and some plants (palm, palm-kernel and coconut oils).

It's also wise to limit the amount of cholesterol you get directly from foods. Cholesterol is found in any animal product, but is particularly high in egg yolks and organ meats. The daily recommended limit is 300 milligrams (one yolk has 275).

USDA recommendations call for no more than 30 percent of daily calories to come from fats. Since fat is more than twice as high in calories as protein or carbohydrates (9 calories per gram versus 4), that restricts you to only a few tablespoons daily. The nutritional guidelines also say that no more than 10 percent of these calories should be from saturated fat. The unsaturated fats—canola, corn, cottonseed, olive, peanut, rapeseed, safflower, soybean and sunflower oils—should make up the remaining 20 percent. Unsaturated fats don't harm the heart, and most will actually lower cholesterol. However, they're still high in calories and should be limited if you want to lose weight.

One type of unsaturated fat that is proving beneficial to those with arthritis is eicosapentaenoic acid (EPA), found in cold-water fish and seafood such as mackerel, lake trout, herring, salmon, oysters and tuna. Researchers believe that this fatty acid affects the production of prostaglandins, and so interferes with the inflammation process; several studies in animals and humans have borne this out. Further research is needed to determine whether eating more of these types of seafood—or taking fish-oil capsules (see "Nutritional Supplements" below)—will improve arthritis in the long term. In addition, cold-water seafood is also high in omega-3 fatty acids; these substances have been proven to protect against heart disease, a known risk to those who have arthritis.

• **Avoid too much sugar.** Sugar provides no nutrition, just calories. Even if you're underweight, you should not rely on sweets to fill most of your daily calorie needs—that road leads to malnutrition. Sugar also raises blood sugar rapidly and drops it just as quickly; this can depress your system, leaving you vulnerable to fatigue and pain.

• **Eat foods with adequate starch and fiber.** Some medications can cause constipation, as can too little exercise, since exercise naturally helps move food through the bowels. Complex carbohydrates should make up the bulk of your diet—60 percent or more. They not only improve digestion but are also high in nutrients. The richest sources are whole cereals, such as wheat and wheat bran, brown rice, corn, barley, rye and millet; legumes, including white beans, cowpeas, chickpeas, kidney beans, lentils, limas, navy beans, peanuts and peas; root vegetables like potatoes, carrots, parsnips, turnips and sweet potatoes; fresh fruits, especially berries and apples; and vegetables such as broccoli, brussels sprouts, cabbage, greens and squash (summer and winter varieties).

• **Avoid too much sodium.** Water retention is a side effect of several arthritis drugs (see Chapter 7). In addition, about 25 to 50 percent of gout sufferers also have high blood pressure, a condition linked to high-salt diets. The USDA guidelines advise limiting salt to 1,100 to 3,300 milligrams a day—equal to about one-half to one-and-a-half teaspoonfuls. You'd be better off shaking the salt habit completely; the body does require some sodium, but can get what it needs naturally from most foods. (You only need to increase salt intake after prolonged, intense exercise, when the body loses a great deal of sodium through sweat.) Beware of processed foods, which often use large amounts of salt as a preservative.

• **If you drink alcoholic beverages, do so in moderation.** In the case of gout, alcohol seems to stimulate purine production; beer also contains yeast, which is high in purines. In addition, most arthritis drugs don't mix with alcohol. Remember, too, that alcohol is a depressant and can hamper your ability to cope with your condition. Current recommendations suggest no more than one drink per day for women, two for men. However, avoid alcoholic beverages altogether if you need to lose weight; they're high in calories and low in nutrition.

Nutritional Supplements

Medical researchers are aware that some types of arthritis are linked with deficiencies in certain nutrients. However, these conditions are a *result* of the disease or the drugs used to treat them, rather than the *cause* of illness. Taking large doses of vitamins or minerals will not cure arthritis—and may worsen it. Too much of a nutrient can be as damaging as too little. Unless advised otherwise by your doctor, you shouldn't take a daily supplement that contains more than 100 percent of the Recommended Dietary Allowances (RDAs) for any vitamin or mineral.

It has been noted that rheumatoid arthritis patients have lower than normal levels of histidine (an amino acid) and vitamin C. Supplements of these nutrients helped the deficiency, but brought little direct improvement of the arthritis.

Chronic diseases like rheumatoid arthritis often result in a type of anemia caused by the inability of iron to enter red blood cells and manufacture hemoglobin. Unfortunately, unlike the anemia brought on by iron deficiency, this condition cannot be helped by increasing iron in the diet or by supplementing. Also be aware that arthritis drugs such as NSAIDs can trigger gastrointestinal bleeding, creating another type of anemia that can be eliminated by raising iron levels. Your doctor can test you to determine which condition you have.

RA patients are also low in B6 (pyroxidine). One researcher showed that 100 milligrams of this B vitamin a day helped somewhat in arthritis of the hands and carpal tunnel syndrome; however, these results have not been duplicated.

Another B vitamin, niacin, was touted as an arthritis reliever in the wake of a 1950s study. However, the poorly controlled research has never been confirmed. In addition, too much niacin can increase uric acid in the blood, leading to gout.

Vitamin C has a role in the creation of collagen. In animals, high doses have been shown to slow down erosion of cartilage in osteoarthritis. More study is needed to see whether this holds true for human subjects.

As noted in Chapter 7, corticosteroids draw calcium from bones. In order to prevent osteoporosis, the bone-thinning disease, your doctor will probably advise you to take a calcium supplement, such as calcium carbonate. You may also need to take vitamin D, which helps the body absorb calcium. You should make an effort to add more calcium to your diet naturally, through milk, yogurt, low-fat cheeses, and vegetables such as kale, greens and broccoli. Salmon and sardines, with bones, are also high in calcium. Another hint: Swallow a calcium supplement with milk (the lactose helps your stomach absorb the calcium better) or orange juice (vitamin C does the same).

As mentioned above, fish oils that contain eicosapentaenoic acid (EPA) show some promise in reducing symptoms of rheumatoid arthritis, but have yet to be conclusively studied in humans. One experiment with RA patients did include an EPA supplement in a high-unsaturated-fat diet; morning stiffness, as well as the number of joints affected, was reduced. Another study reported that high doses of fish oil taken daily, without any other change in diet, improved some cases of RA. At this point, dosage amounts that are safe and effective have not been determined, and it's not clear that taking fish-oil capsules is better than getting EPA through its natural source, seafood. High doses of fish oil also have side effects, including diarrhea and blood thinning.

Elimination Diets

Diets that leave out a particular food or food group have long been whispered as a "cure" for arthritis. Research has not been able to back up these claims consistently. Food allergies have been mentioned as a trigger to arthritis, and some substances do seem to provoke symptoms in some people. For instance, eating black walnuts induced knee inflammation in one sufferer. In human and animal studies, alfalfa seeds and sprouts brought on a lupus-like condition. In one case of rheumatoid arthritis it was reported that dairy products caused the condition to worsen within twenty-four hours.

However, these types of reactions show up in a very small portion of patients, rarely hold up in random testing and so cannot be applied to the general population. Food allergies can't be found in most arthritis patients, and they definitely don't cause the disease. In addition, trying to find out what you might be allergic to is tedious and nearly impossible, as you must eliminate specific foods one by one, for weeks at a time.

Several elimination diets have become well known. The Childers diet suggests avoiding all substances in the nightshade family—tomatoes, white potatoes, eggplant, bell peppers (including paprika) and tobacco. The Dong diet stresses fish and vegetables, and advocates avoiding red meat, dairy products, fruit, alcohol and preservatives. The Airola diet starts with a period of fasting before following a vegetarian regimen (it includes dairy products; little salt, sugar or white flour; and no alcohol, tobacco, coffee or tea). Raw fruits and vegetables are the staples of the Warmbrand diet, which eliminates high-fat cheese, meat, fish, eggs and refined foods. Again, under scientific investigation, only a few arthritis patients benefited from such diets.

Fasting (ingesting only vegetable and fruit juices and water) and very-low-calorie diets have reduced arthritis symptoms temporarily for some people. However, these drastic restrictions can be dangerous to the heart and other bodily systems if continued for longer than a few weeks or months.

If all other therapies fail or if you experience a marked change in symptoms after you eat certain foods, you may be tempted to try one of these diets. There is a chance one may work for you. However, don't try any diet as a substitute for your usual arthritis treatment, and never go on any diet without consulting your doctor. The danger is that you might eliminate a food that's vital to your health, and without it you may do more harm than good for your arthritis.

CHAPTER 10

Exploring the "Alternatives"

Even with the various therapies your doctor has prescribed for your arthritis, you may become discouraged at times. Some medications require time to take effect. Exercise and joint protection techniques must be followed consistently to be most beneficial. You may wonder whether there's a quicker, easier way to get relief. There will always be someone who will tell you that there is—and who will be happy to sell it to you.

"Alternative" treatments for arthritis abound. Many are outright health frauds, produced to take advantage of the frustration often faced by those with chronic illnesses. Some are based on folk remedies that were popular before modern medicines were developed. Of these, a few have been shown to have real merit and are now a part of conventional arthritis therapy. Others may yet prove to have value, but without well-controlled, long-term studies there's no way of knowing how effective or safe they are. In addition, promising new medicines and methods, still in the research stage, become public knowledge through newspaper and television reports and are promoted before their safety and worth have been fully tested. Any remedy that's not available through your own physician should be greeted with skepticism.

At some point in the course of their disease, about 90 percent of arthritis patients will try such an unproven remedy. In the United States every year, between $1 billion and $2 billion are spent on questionable treatments. But financial cost is the least concern: The price you pay may be your health.

Dangerous Deceptions

When it comes to unproven remedies, the phrase "There's no harm in trying" does not apply. Besides wasting money, they waste time—time better spent on treatments that are known to work. When you delay in seeking out a proven therapy, you allow the disease to progress. Alternative treatments give a false hope of a cure, and when they don't work, you may be too discouraged or depressed to get real help. And even more dangerous, some of these products contain ingredients that are harmful or that could trigger a deadly allergic reaction.

Why are so many arthritis sufferers drawn to unproven remedies? These products are highly publicized by the companies that make them, with claims that are too good to be true. You may even know someone who has tried one and swears by it. Often quack cures do seem to work, though scientifically they should not. In some cases, improvement can be traced to the *placebo effect*. This mind-over-matter phenomenon is well known to research scientists: Some studies have shown that if given a capsule that contains nothing more potent than sugar (the placebo), about 30 to 40 percent of patients, suffering from all types of illnesses, will feel better—at least temporarily. They believe it will work, expect it to work or want it to work so badly that their bodies respond. (When developing new drugs, a placebo is often given to a portion of the subjects—known as the "control" group—to check whether it's the experimental medication or just the power of positive thinking that is responsible for the patient's improvement.) However, the effect of a placebo-like product rarely brings a lasting change in the condition. But in the meantime, the unproven remedy may be enthusiastically endorsed by those who have tried it.

Coincidence is another reason for the success of some unconventional treatments. As you know, arthritis is a disease of unpredictable ups and downs. If you take any substance long enough, it's likely that a "cure" will take place eventually—when the flare-up would naturally subside. If you swallow a remedy just before the start of a typical remission, you might be convinced that the product did the trick.

Recently, chemical analyses of some "natural" herbal mixtures have revealed where they get their miraculous powers: They contain doses of the same corticosteroids or NSAIDs used in conventional arthritis therapy. (This is discussed further in "Folk Remedies," below.) They may work—but you're not getting what you paid for. What's worse, you may suffer side effects that won't be monitored by a doctor.

Common Alternatives

Several types of health therapies that do not have the approval of most medical professionals are still well known and widely used. Some of these alternative medicines have relieved certain arthritic symptoms for a short time, and may be an option if you can't take drugs.

Lower back pain may be helped through a chiropractor's "adjustment" of the spine. Chiropractors are not M.D.'s, and are still not officially accepted by the American Medical Association, but many people get relief from these practitioners. (Some feel worse.) The chiropractic technique—which may include massage, ultrasound or electrical stimulation as well—won't permanently improve your joints. However, if it's covered by your health insurance plan and your doctor approves, you may want to try chiropractic to ease pain temporarily.

Popular in Europe, homeopathy is sought out by many Americans who prefer a holistic (whole body) approach to healing and want to avoid the side effects of conventional medicines. In this practice, developed over two hundred years ago, patients are given "remedies" containing tiny amounts of animal, plant or mineral substances; each dose is specifically matched to an individual's group of symptoms. Homeopathic practitioners believe that these substances, which if given in higher doses would actually re-create the same symptoms, act like vaccines to stimulate the body's immune system to eliminate the disease itself. In the case of arthritis, homeopaths do not claim to cure the condition, only to relieve some of its symptoms. (Many homeopaths are also medical doctors who prescribe more traditional therapies when immediate care is needed.) However, homeopathic remedies are not considered scientifically sound—they are so highly diluted that they would hold few or none of the substance's original molecules. Anyone taking homeopathic therapy must follow strict guidelines for dosing and lifestyle changes, and it may take several tries to find the "right" remedy. Overall, homepathy has not proved to be better than a placebo and requires as much commitment as any conventional therapy, though many people find comfort in the personal care given by a homeopath.

A few trials have studied acupuncture as a pain-relief measure in arthritis. It has been shown to help some rheumatoid arthritis patients, though not those with osteoarthritis. Why is not clear; it may work as a placebo or by triggering the release of endorphins. In this ancient Chinese therapy, very thin steel needles are inserted at specific sites in the body (which may or may not be near arthritic joints), and then rotated by hand, or a low electrical current is applied. Treatments are repeated as often as once a week. TENS (transcutaneous electrical nerve stimulation, discussed in Chapter 6) can offer results similar to that achieved by electrical acupuncture but more safely and conveniently, with less expense and discomfort.

Reflexology, the latest in faddish "manipulation" techniques, holds that each system of the body is connected to a specific pressure point located on your feet. While there is nothing that connects this theory to reality, if you find a foot massage relaxing, reflexology may have some benefit for you.

Folk Remedies: Wisdom or Quackery?

Many medicines that are in wide use today got their start as folk remedies. For instance, as mentioned in Chapter 7, early arthritis patients took willow-tree bark, now known to be the source of salicylate, an effective arthritis treatment. Gold salts were dispensed for forty years before their medical benefits were verified. However, dosing yourself with willow-tree bark or gold is still risky unless you're under a doctor's supervision.

Questionable treatments for arthritis have been circulating for centuries. Some have a basis in medical science; others are pure quackery. Overall, none is more effective than conventional therapies, and a few can be harmful. The most common concoctions, and their usefulness, are discussed below.

Venoms. Strangely enough, research has shown that some venoms do reduce inflammation in rheumatoid arthritis. The reason: Bee and ant venom contain chemicals that stimulate your adrenal glands to produce their own corticosteroids. (Snake venoms have not been studied.) Unless you plan on becoming a beekeeper, though, the cost of venom equivalent to about two dozen bee stings (the amount needed to be beneficial) or the pain from the real thing hardly makes this an attractive treatment. A more serious concern, though, is triggering a deadly allergic reaction, a risk that increases with each exposure to venom.

Herbs and extracts. Plant remedies seem to be formulated on the notion that the arthritis sufferer is missing a vital nutrient, which just isn't true. Yucca and aloe vera are traditional "healing herbs," but not for arthritis. Some products are made from alfalfa, which actually triggers flare-ups in some people. Extracts of seaweed, seawater and the green-lipped mussel are also promoted, and useless, for arthritis treatment. Specimens of Chinese herbal medicines, such as Chuei-Fong-Gen-Wan and Tsai-Tsa-Wan, were found to be laced with prednisone, dexamethasone, indomethacin and other known arthritis drugs—which should only be taken under a doctor's care. Other chemically analyzed products proved to be contaminated by other toxic substances, like lead.

Devices. Steer clear of any gadget that its maker claims reverses arthritis through radio waves, electrons, magnetic fields, or some other scientific-sounding jargon. Vibrating chairs and beds, perhaps developed with the idea of massaging away pain, can instead irritate inflamed joints further. Wearing mitts or bracelets containing uranium, even sitting in an abandoned uranium mine, have been touted as "irradiating" arthritis, but they give off little or no radioactivity—or benefit. Copper bracelets were worn by the ancient Greeks as a treatment for aches. (More recently, early treatments of rheumatoid arthritis with copper salts caused some improvement, but also many serious side effects.) Still, it's doubtful, even if the copper from a bracelet could be absorbed through the skin, that it would affect arthritis.

Lotions and ointments. You may have heard that applying motor oil or brake fluid will "lubricate" joints. You may see arthritis liniments, containing methol or camphor, for sale. These remedies usually create a tingling or warmth that can distract from pain and may have a use in some arthritis cases, but don't expect much more than that. Some may list salicylate, other drugs or vitamins as ingredients; however, these substances have no effect on joints when rubbed on the skin. Another well-advertised ointment, dimethyl sulfoxide (DMSO), does penetrate more deeply and has shown to help inflammation for some types of arthritis. Though an impure form is prescribed as a painkiller in veterinary medicine, DMSO has not been approved for human use by the Food and Drug Administration, which did not find enough evidence in the drug's favor. Unfortunately, many people have traveled to clinics outside the United States in search of DMSO, only to be fooled into buying potions that contain corticosteroids, phenylbutazone or other potent drugs.

Miscellaneous therapies. Several experimental drugs as well as combinations of sex hormones have been publicized as being beneficial in treating some forms of arthritis. Unfortunately, this notoriety creates a premature demand— which often continues long after careful research shows that a remedy is ineffective or has dangerous side effects.

Be wary of any such product sold only by sources outside this country; not only might they be illegal, they cannot be guaranteed to contain the ingredients advertised.

There are plenty of other, quainter, remedies that have survived over the centuries: being buried up to the neck in horse manure, standing naked under a full moon. But besides taking your mind off your arthritis briefly and giving your neighbors something to talk about, they're no substitute for conventional arthritis therapies.

Buyer Beware

Before you try any unproven remedy or alternative therapy that you've read or heard about, discuss it with your physician. He or she will be able to steer you clear of useless or dangerous treatments. Your doctor may even suggest an alternative treatment if the method has not been widely tested but has been shown to be beneficial to some patients. If your condition is not improving with conventional therapies, your doctor may also agree to allow you to use an unproven remedy as a last resort, as long as it is not inherently harmful.

Even without your doctor's help, you can spot a health fraud. Bogus products generally give themselves away by the way they're advertised or promoted, and by what they do or *don't* tell you on their labels. Your suspicions should be aroused by any one of the following signs.

• **It sounds too good to be true.** Most likely it's neither good nor true. Often these products promise to help not only all types of arthritis, but high blood pressure, depression and a host of other ailments—in the hope that you'll be more willing to hand over your money for two cures for the price of one.

• **A cure is offered.** As of yet, arthritis has no cure. A product that claims otherwise is meant to appeal to the desperate and the chronically ill. If it were an actual cure, everyone would know about it.

• **The product is advertised as a "secret formula," or its ingredients are "special," "exclusive" or "breakthrough."** In addition, the actual contents may not be listed on the label. Why are the manufacturers so anxious to conceal what goes into their product? Legitimate scientists are willing to share their discoveries. Also be skeptical of the word "natural," which is meant to be synonymous with "harmless": Many plants, herbs or other substances are natural, but also poisonous.

• **The label does not list side effects or explain how to use the product or for how long.** Should the remedy be taken before or after meals? Is it safe for children or for adults with other health problems? Can relief be expected immediately or over several days? These are questions that any consumer should ask. If you can't find the answers packaged along with the product, the manufacturer isn't concerned about its customers' health.

• **Personal testimonials are offered as proof.** If you see the names, pictures and "true stories" of individuals who say a product worked for them, you may be more inclined to try it yourself. But the testimony of a handful of people is no proof that the remedy will work for the majority of arthritis sufferers. Of course, you also have no way of verifying the quotations or faces used.

• **The claims are based on an attack on traditional medicine.** For instance, a manufacturer may bill its product as "the remedy your doctor won't tell you about" or "doesn't know about." These makers promote fear or distrust of the medical establishment for their own gain.

• **No scientifically investigated proof is presented, or only one study is cited.** A remedy should be thoroughly tested before it's offered to the public. In scientific research, the most impartial way to gather evidence is through a double-blind study: Neither the subject nor the researcher knows whether the subject was given the experimental treatment or a placebo. This research method helps prove whether the remedy alone—and not the expectations of the subject or the researcher—influenced the results. Sometimes one study does seem to show that a treatment is worthwhile, but similar tests conducted by other scientists don't confirm this finding. It may be that other factors present during the first experiment brought about the results. If the results cannot be consistently repeated, the treatment can be assumed to have no value.

• **The product is only available by mail order or phone, through ads in newspapers, magazines, books or on television.** A successful treatment would be accessible to doctors and would be reviewed in a number of medical journals. In addition, any company that has only a post office box or a telephone number or works out of an obscure town or foreign country obviously wants to make it difficult for dissatisfied customers to track it down.

You may assume that any remedy advertised or for sale on a store shelf has some value—or else why wouldn't state or federal authorities have made them illegal? Unfortunately, agencies such as the Food and Drug Administration can't crack down on all fraudulent products—there are just too many, and often the companies that produce them operate for a short while, then take the money and run. Some get around the law by not making specific claims that could get them into trouble.

You can protect yourself by learning as much as you can about arthritis so that you know how it can be treated realistically. We hope that *Living with Arthritis* has given you that background, and that you'll investigate on your own and keep up with the latest research developments through reliable sources, such as medical journals, the Arthritis Foundation and your doctor.

CHAPTER 11

In the Future

Not so long ago, if you had arthritis, your chances of leading a relatively normal life were far less predictable. Conditions such as rheumatoid arthritis were often crippling, and others, like lupus, could be fatal. Fortunately, thanks to recent improvements in physical therapy, pain management and medications, these dire consequences are almost things of the past.

Despite these successes, though, medical researchers have not given up their mission to eliminate arthritis entirely, while in the meantime finding the safest and most reliable treatments. Helping in their search are new technologies that allow them a closer look at the way genes and the immune system work. Clues to the causes of specific conditions are being investigated continually, and more and more breakthroughs are reported each year.

Genetic Research

The first step toward curing any disease is uncovering the cause. When scientists can't find a virus, bacteria or other obvious triggering agent, they look for genetic markers—a gene or group of genes common to those who have the same form of arthritis. As discussed in Chapter 2, we know that rheumatoid arthritis is associated with the genes HLA-DR4 and sometimes HLA-DR1. HLA-B27 has been detected in about 95 percent of cases of ankylosing spondylitis, 60 percent of cases of Reiter's syndrome and about 40 to 50 percent of psoriatic arthritis cases. In a rare form of osteoarthritis, a genetic defect has been detected in the protein known as type II collagen, an essential component of cartilage. In many cases, though, it is still unknown whether the genetic marker itself plays an active role in the development of the disease or whether it's merely a signpost pointing to a particular area on the chromosome.

One gene rarely acts alone—usually two or three genes are involved in creating a predisposition to an illness. You must get a set of each from both your mother and your father; inheriting only some of the genes may determine whether your arthritis will be less severe. In some cases, faulty genes express themselves only if triggered by an outside force, such as an infection, which may begin the disease process but is gone and can no longer be detected by the time arthritis symptoms develop. (For instance, gene amplification of the synovial fluid of some patients with Reiter's syndrome has revealed "footprints" of chlamydia, a sexually transmitted infection.) All these components, and how they interact, need to be known in order for researchers to come up with a surefire solution to arthritis.

Other genes involved in the immune system affecting T cells are also under investigation. As you may remember from Chapter 2, these cells are lymphocytes, a form of white blood cell, which can help destroy invading organisms and also regulate other parts of the immune system. T cells named CD4 have been found in tissue affected by rheumatoid arthritis and lupus, and are thought to be the major contributor to these diseases. Supporting this theory is the discovery that these conditions improve in some patients who have arthritis after they are also stricken with AIDS, a usually fatal disease that is known to wipe out CD4 cells. In ankylosing spondylitis and other spondyloarthropathies, CD8 T cells may be at work. It has also been noted that these diseases in AIDS patients become worse, because the lack of CD4 cells allows CD8 to multiply.

Scientists can also try to confirm the suspected causes of arthritis by attempting to "manufacture" the diseases in the laboratory. For instance, when researchers at the University of Texas Southwestern Medical School in Dallas recently inserted human HLA-B27 genes into the developing eggs of rats, the rodents developed inflammation of the large joints and spine, scaly skin and diarrhea—symptoms similar to those of the spondyloarthropathies. These animal models will also be helpful in further research—for instance, exposing them to an infection to see whether it triggers disease in animals genetically susceptible to arthritis.

What happens after specific genetic markers like HLA genes or T cell subtypes have been identified? Scientists can then modify, eliminate or interfere with them. One way is to remove the disease-causing gene, or add a protective gene. Such gene therapy is already a reality: In a National Institutes of Health test case, a young girl with a rare immune-deficiency disorder was given white blood cells inserted with the gene that her own cells were missing. Boosted by these doctored cells, her white blood cells began manufacturing the enzymes necessary to prevent her immune system from being destroyed. Right now, this isn't a permanent solution (treatments must be repeated), but it is on the road to a cure.

Understanding the Immune System

For autoimmune disorders like rheumatoid arthritis, understanding the immune process is crucial to treating the disease. How the body's "defense system" works to bring about inflammation was explained in Chapter 2; however, much about the immune system is still a mystery. Recently biologists discovered a "second switch" that turns on the immune response. It seems that T cells need two signals to begin to attack foreign material in the body: First, protein fragments from the antigens must be displayed on other white blood cell surfaces so that the T cells can recognize them; then the same cells must push other proteins, called B7 molecules, to their surfaces to stimulate proteins on the surfaces of the T cells, called CD28. This final step tells the T cells to divide, multiply and kill off the invaders. Without the second signal, the immune system will not react to the invading organism. Research is now under way to see whether B7 protein can be disarmed to prevent T cells from swinging into action and destroying the body's own tissues.

Other research is exploring why the immune system malfunctions in the first place. One theory is called "molecular mimicry": Bacteria or a virus may produce proteins similar to those found in joint tissue. The infection starts the immune reaction, the "bugs" are eliminated, but the body continues to attack the similar substance still present. This connection seems to be supported by a 1976 report in the *Annals of Internal Medicine:* In an "experiment of Nature," about half the sailors on board a U.S. Navy vessel developed dysentery after infection with *Shigella* (a bacteria that causes severe diarrhea). In a follow-up of these men, 10 percent had gone on to develop Reiter's syndrome; 80 percent of those afflicted were found to have the HLA-B27 gene, which may be responsible for confusing normal tissue substances with whatever has been left by the bacteria.

Hormones can also affect the immune system, and their roles, too, are being explored. Lupus, which is more common in females, has been hormonally manipulated in some strains of mice that have been bred to be susceptible to the disease: Giving these mice the male hormone androgen and suppressing the production of the female hormone estrogen has been shown to prevent the development of lupus. (Unfortunately, the side effects of this hormone treatment are unacceptable in human patients.) In more recent studies, animals injected with a compound called transforming growth-factor beta (TGF-beta) had less inflammation, perhaps because the hormone suppressed the signal for immune cells to gather. In addition, TGF-beta and insulin-like growth factor 1 regulate the repair and maintenance of cartilage, which is abnormal in osteoarthritis; in the future it may be possible to stimulate cells into producing these growth factors when and where they are needed.

Better Medicines

Many medications used in arthritis are like blasting away with a shotgun: The disease is hit, but so are normal bystander cells, which is why the drugs have side effects. Pinpointing which HLA genes or T cells are involved in each type of arthritis would allow researchers to formulate a therapy that would target only these disease-causing cells.

Until then, though, research continues toward creating treatments as reliably effective as those for gout. With 37 million arthritis sufferers as potential customers, drug makers as well as medical scientists have an interest in developing new medications and are now working on about two hundred potential arthritis remedies. Most are variations on the NSAIDs. Some of these are already available in other countries, and are being tested or are awaiting approval in the United States. The goal is to find medicines for people who cannot tolerate those now in use, and also to improve disease-fighting ability and reduce the side effects of current drugs.

Interleuken-1 and interferon, two drugs used in cancer therapy, may eventually be used to treat severe rheumatoid arthritis. These substances are known to block cytokines, hormone-like substances released by T cells to provoke inflammation. Both interleuken-1 and interferon are chemicals found naturally in the body and are involved in the immune process.

In addition, drugs are being developed that block the nervous system's effect on the pain of the inflammatory response. The substance that makes chili peppers hot—capsaicin—also seems to get in the way of the nervous-system proteins that set off joint pain.

Birth-control pills may have a place in arthritis therapy.

It has been noted that women who take oral contraceptives are less likely to have rheumatoid arthritis. The Pill contains hormones that mimic pregnancy, which naturally improves RA. Studies are now under way to determine whether oral contraceptives reduce the overall risk or just delay the onset of RA.

Advances in Surgery

Joint replacement has become almost routine surgery over the past twenty years, and it continues to improve. Some of the latest innovations are not available everywhere, but the hope is that they soon will be.

Computer imaging has made it possible to custom-design artificial joints for each individual, rather than rely on standard models. Closely matched to your own joint in size and shape, the design is then used for computer-guided construction of the prosthesis. The result is a more natural, easier range of movement.

Replacement of knees and hips has always been tricky because these joints must be precisely positioned to naturally bear the weight and stress of walking, bending, standing and sitting. Advancements in measuring the force and pressure all along the joint surface may ensure the success of future knee and hip replacements.

Some specialized surgical hospitals are testing "component" joints. These are composed of separate pieces that can be replaced as each wears out, rather than having to remove the entire artificial joint. This use of these joints would require less surgery, cutting down on recovery time and complications.

As mentioned in Chapter 8, the "cementless" technique

has shown promise as a natural way to secure a man-made joint, by allowing new bone to grow into the prosthesis.

Nondrug Therapies

Recently, scientists have attempted to remove potentially harmful substances from the circulation by apheresis—from the Greek term meaning "to take by force." In this process, blood is filtered to cleanse it of plasma or lymphocytes. For instance, plasmapheresis—in which withdrawn plasma is replaced by a blood protein called albumin—reduces blood levels of antibodies, immune complexes and other compounds responsible for inflammation. In studies involving RA, benefits lasted for only a few months; the technique may be most helpful for those with severe disease or life-threatening complications. For patients with very active lupus, the results appear to be longer-lasting. So far, however, these procedures are too expensive, impractical and vulnerable to complications for widespread use; they also require that the patient take immunosuppressant drugs, which have their own share of dangerous side effects.

Total lymphoid irradiation (TLI), a technique used for the past twenty-five years in Hodgkin's disease, has been tested as an alternative to cytotoxic drugs for RA patients who did not respond to other therapies. In TLI, lymph nodes are bombarded with radiation to suppress the production of inflammation-causing lymphocytes. Major improvements were reported to last for one to two years. The technique also seems to help lupus that involves kidney damage. However, side effects limit its use to only the most serious cases, though it's possible that TLI could be made safer eventually.

Radiation synovectomy is a popular treatment for RA in Europe, and tests here have shown positive results. In this procedure, radioactive isotopes are injected in the synovium to eradicate diseased tissue. Concerns about exposure to radiation and the possibility of isotopes leaking from joints to other parts of the body still must be answered.

A highly experimental therapy that has had success for certain other immune-system ailments has been tested recently on a small group of RA patients. In this method, called extracorporeal photochemotherapy (ECP), the patient takes a light-activated drug; T cells incorporate the drug, then are removed from the patient and treated with light, and then reinjected into the patient. The immune system wipes out these cells and prevents other similar T cells, which might cause the autoimmmine disease, from multiplying. In its preliminary trial at Yale University, ECP reduced joint swelling and tenderness in four of the seven patients—results encouraging enough for researchers to begin a larger study.

Many other areas in the prevention and treatment of arthritis are being investigated, and may someday provide the key to unlocking the mysteries surrounding most forms of arthritis. Keep up to date on the latest breakthroughs that affect your condition; some of the organizations and publications in the next chapter can help in your continuing education. In the meantime, though, following your own program of exercise, pain control and drug therapy is your surest guarantee that—despite your arthritis—you will enjoy a long, healthy and active life.

CHAPTER 12

For More Information

General Resources

Organizations

Arthritis Foundation
1314 Spring Street N.W.
Atlanta, GA 30309
(800) 283-7800 or (404) 872-7100

This national nonprofit organization provides extensive information through printed materials, most at no cost, on the individual types of arthritis and treatments, as well as tips for coping with the physical and emotional consequences of the disease. Through its local chapters, in nearly every state, the foundation offers seminars, self-help courses, exercise classes and support groups; referrals for arthritis specialists, therapists and clinics; and guidance in locating government agencies that can help with financial, employment and other concerns. Check your phone book or contact the national headquarters above for the chapter nearest you to obtain publications and find out what services are available in your area.

The Arthritis Society
250 Bloor Street East
Suite 401
Toronto, Ontario M4W 3P2, Canada
(416) 967-1414

Canada's equivalent of the Arthritis Foundation, this organization also offers a variety of informative materials through its many chapters.

National Arthritis and Musculoskeletal and Skin
    Diseases Information Clearinghouse
900 Rockville Pike
Box AMS
Bethesda, MD 20892
(301) 495-4484

Funded by the National Institute of Arthritis, Musculoskeletal and Skin Diseases (NIAMS), this agency will perform a literature search and provide a bibliography on any arthritis topic if requested in writing. The clearinghouse also offers a listing of materials you can send for and data bases for computer searches.

In addition, NIAMS, which is one of the federal National Institutes of Health, supports research at various academic institutions around the country. These Multipurpose Arthritis and Musculoskeletal Diseases Centers may offer education and health services to the public. Contact the center nearest you, listed below in alphabetical order by state, for more information. (Also check with your local university or medical school, which may have

its own specialized arthritis center or can refer you to one
in your area.)

UAB Arthritis Center
429 Tinsley Harrison Towers
Birmingham, AL 35294
(800) 345-6780

W. M. Keck Autoimmune Disease Center
Scripps Clinic and Research Foundation
Department of Molecular and Experimental
  Medicine
10666 North Torrey Pines Road
La Jolla, CA 92037
(619) 455-9100

Division of Rheumatology
University of California School of Medicine
1000 Veteran Avenue
Los Angeles, CA 90024-1670
(310) 825-7991

Stanford Arthritis Center
701 Welch Road, Suite 3301
Palo Alto, CA 94303
(415) 723-5907

University of California School of Medicine
San Francisco General Hospital
1001 Potrero Avenue
Building 30, Room 3300
San Francisco, CA 94110
(415) 821-8189

Division of Rheumatic Diseases
University of Connecticut School of Medicine
263 Farmington Avenue
Farmington, CT 06030-1310
(203) 679-3290

Northwestern University Medical School
Arthritis–Connective Tissue Diseases Division
Ward 3-315
303 East Chicago Avenue
Chicago, IL 60611
(312) 503-8197

Division of Rheumatology
Indiana University School of Medicine
541 Clinical Drive
Indianapolis, IN 46223
(317) 274-4225

Boston University School of Medicine
80 East Concord Street
Boston, MA 02118
(617) 638-4310

Department of Rheumatology
Brigham and Women's Hospital
75 Francis Street
Boston, MA 02115
(617) 732-5325

Division of Rheumatology
University of Michigan Medical School
Taubman Center, Room 3918
1500 East Medical Center Drive
Box 0358

Ann Arbor, MI 48109-0358
(313) 936-5562

Arthritis and Musculoskeletal Diseases Center at the
  Hospital for Special Surgery
535 East 70th Street
New York, NY 10021
(212) 606-1189

Thurston Arthritis Center
School of Medicine, Department of Medicine
Division of Rheumatology and Immunology
University of North Carolina at Chapel Hill
CB 7280
932 Faculty Laboratory Office Building 231H
Chapel Hill, NC 27599-7280
(919) 966-4191

Division of Rheumatology
University Hospitals of Cleveland
2074 Abington Road
Cleveland, OH 44106
(216) 844-3168

Books

Arthritis Foundation (ed.: Irving Kushner, M.D.), *Understanding Arthritis*. New York: Scribner's, 1984.
Fries, James F., M.D., *Arthritis: A Comprehensive Guide to Understanding Your Arthritis*. Reading, MA: Addison-Wesley, 1990.
Lorig, Kate, R.N., Dr. P.H., and James F. Fries, M.D., *The Arthritis Helpbook*. Reading, MA: Addison-Wesley, 1980.

Periodicals

Arthritis Today. A bimonthly publication distributed free to members of the Arthritis Foundation, with a basic contribution of $20.

Accent on Living. P.O. Box 700, Bloomington, IL 61701.

Closer Look. National Information Center for the Handicapped, P.O. Box 1492, Washington, DC 20013.

Mainstream: Magazine of the Able-Disabled. 861 Sixth Avenue, Suite 610, San Diego, CA 92101.

Videotapes

Self-Help with Robin May emphasizes how to use assistive devices in everyday activities. Available from the Arthritis Foundation, New York Chapter, 67 Irving Place, New York, NY 10003; (212) 477-8310.

Living with Arthritis is an hour-long overview of the disease, with descriptions of the services offered by the Arthritis Foundation. *PACE (People with Arthritis Can Exercise)* allows you to continue at home the movements taught in the foundation's PACE classes. *PEP (Pool Exercise Program)* outlines a water workout to improve range of motion. All available from the Arthritis Foundation; contact your local chapter.

Specialized Organizations

Ankylosing Spondylitis Association
511 North La Cienega, Box 216
Los Angeles, CA 90048
(800) 777-8189 or (310) 652-0609

This nonprofit group provides education and support for AS patients through local chapters and contacts. A newsletter is sent to members quarterly.

American Juvenile Arthritis Organization
1314 Spring Street N.W.
Atlanta, GA 30309
(800) 283-7800 or (404) 872-7100

A division of the Arthritis Foundation, the AJAO organizes services such as workshops and recreational activities for young arthritis sufferers and their families through local chapters.

Lupus Foundation of America
4 Research Place, Suite 180
Rockville, MD 20850-3226
(800) 558-0121; in Spanish (800) 558-0231

This national voluntary health organization offers patient information, physician referrals, support groups and other services through its local chapters. Members also receive *Lupus News*, a triannual newsletter.

National Psoriasis Foundation
Suite 210
6443 Southwest Beaverton Highway
Portland, OR 97221
(503) 297-1545

This nonprofit foundation publishes educational material and supports research. Members are sent a bulletin six times a year.

Scleroderma Research Foundation
Box 200

Columbus, NJ 08022
(609) 261 2200

This nonprofit foundation offers support and education to scleroderma patients.

Sjögren's Syndrome Foundation, Inc.
382 Main Street
Port Washington, NY 11050
(516) 767-2866

Through local chapters and contacts across the country, this foundation offers educational materials and organizes support groups. Members receive a monthly newsletter.

United Scleroderma Foundation, Inc.
P.O. Box 399
Watsonville, CA 95077-0399
(800) 722-HOPE

With twenty-six chapters in the United States and one in Canada, this organization sponsors workshops for patients and their families. Published information is also available.

Exercise and Joint Protection

American Occupational Therapy Association
1383 Piccard Drive
P.O. Box 1725
Rockville, MD 20849-1725
(301) 948-9626

Write to the association's Direct Mail Department for a list of accredited occupational therapists.

American Physical Therapy Association
1111 North Fairfax Street
Alexandria, VA 22314
(703) 684-2782

Call or write for a list of accredited physical therapists.

Aquatics Programs; PACE (People with Arthritis Can Exercise)

The Arthritis Foundation presents exercise classes through its chapters. The Aquatics Programs are often cosponsored by local YMCAs or other groups. PACE programs last about six to eight weeks, and exercises can be continued at home with a videotape. The foundation also has Joint Effort classes for those with very limited movement; exercises are performed while seated. However, none of these programs replaces whatever exercises have been mapped out for you by your doctor or therapist.

Guide to Independent Living

Prepared by the Arthritis Health Professions Section of the Arthritis Foundation, this spiral-bound book catalogs hundreds of products that aid in joint protection and provides general suggestions for adapting implements and living areas for your comfort. Included, too, are nearly four hundred mail-order sources for the items mentioned, and additional resources for each topic, such as grooming, travel, meal preparation and recreation. The guide is available through your local Arthritis Foundation chapter for $9.95.

Pain Management

The American Pain Society
5700 Old Orchard Road
Skokie, IL 60077
(708) 966-5595

The society publishes a directory of accredited pain clinics.

Commission on Accreditation of Rehabilitation
   Facilities
101 North Wilmot Road
Suite 500
Tucson, AZ 85711
(602) 748-1212

Send a stamped, self-addressed envelope for a list of accredited pain treatment centers in your area. A directory of centers across the country is also available for $25.

International Pain Foundation
909 Northeast 43rd Street, Suite 306
Seattle, WA 98105
(206) 547-2157

The foundation, affiliated with the International Association for the Study of Pain, publishes the research journal *Pain* and offers information on pain management techniques to the public.

Glossary

ANA: see *antinuclear antibodies*.

ankylosing spondylitis: a chronic disease that causes inflammation of the spine and joints. Affected bones can sometimes grow together (fuse).

antibody: proteins produced by the body to combat a foreign substance or organism such as a virus or bacteria.

antigen: a foreign substance or organism that, when it enters the body, triggers the production of antibodies to destroy it.

anti-inflammatory drugs: medications that combat or reduce inflammation, including aspirin, ibuprofen and the corticosteroids.

antimalarial drugs: slow-acting medications derived from quinine, a substance found in the bark of the Peruvian cinchona tree. Originally a treatment for malaria, they are also prescribed for rheumatoid arthritis, lupus, discoid lupus and juvenile rheumatoid arthritis.

antinuclear antibodies (ANA): antibodies in the blood that attach to the nuclei of cells. Due to abnormality in the immune system, these substances are found in patients with lupus, Sjögren's syndrome and scleroderma, and in some cases of juvenile and rheumatoid arthritis.

arthritis: a general term that covers more than 100 diseases characterized by inflammation of the joints.

arthrodesis: surgically immobilizing a joint so that the bones grow together (fuse).

arthrography: an X ray of a joint, after the injection of a radiological dye, to look for damage to cartilage and synovium.

arthroplasty: rebuilding or replacement of a damaged joint.

arthroscopy: examination or surgery of joint tissues through a periscope-like device inserted into the joint.

AS: see *ankylosing spondylitis.*

aspirin: a medication that reduces inflammation by interfering with the formation of prostaglandins; used to treat several types of arthritis. Though nonprescription, this drug can cause serious side effects (usually ulcers) if used in large doses over prolonged periods.

autoimmune disorder: a disease that occurs when the body produces antibodies that attack its own tissues; linked to rheumatoid arthritis, lupus and Sjögren's syndrome.

B cell: a type of white blood cell that manufactures antibodies.

biopsy: removal of small amount of tissue from the muscle, skin, kidney, artery or joint so that it can be examined for signs of inflammation or autoimmune response.

Bouchard's nodes: a bony growth, or spur, that forms in the middle joints of the fingers; a symptom of osteoarthritis.

bursa: a fluid-filled, membrane-lined sac near a joint that acts as a shock absorber and lubricant among bones, ligaments and tendons.

bursitis: inflammation of a bursa.

cartilage: tough but elastic tissue that connects and covers bone ends, supporting and cushioning a joint.

chronic: said of a condition that lasts a long time or returns frequently.

collagen: a fibrous protein found in cartilage, ligaments and bones.

complement system: a group of proteins involved in the immune reaction. Low levels in the blood may indicate lupus.

computed tomography: a method of X-raying the body that produces a cross-sectional image of the area being examined.

connective tissue: material that supports and binds together other tissues and organs; usually thought of as cartilage, ligaments, muscles, skin and tendons.

corticosteroids: a group of powerful synthetic drugs similar to the natural hormones cortisone and hydrocortisone that reduces inflammation. Large doses and prolonged use lead to severe side effects.

creatinine: a waste product of the body. High levels in the blood may indicate kidney damage.

cryotherapy: using cold to relieve pain.

cytotoxic drugs: potent, slow-acting medications that halt the uncontrolled growth of cells in cancer treatment and prevent the rejection of the donor organ in transplants; sometimes used to control inflammation in severe rheumatoid arthritis, lupus, polymyositis, psoriatic arthritis and vasculitis.

dermatomyositis: a form of arthritis in which inflammation attacks muscles, accompanied by a skin rash on the face or over joints.

discoid lupus: a form of lupus with less serious complications, usually affecting the skin only.

erythrocyte sedimentation rate: also called ESR or sed rate, the measure of how quickly red blood cells settle to the bottom of a blood-filled glass tube. Used as a diagnostic test, ESR indicates whether, or how much, inflammation is present.

fibromyalgia: a chronic condition with symptoms similar to arthritis—aching pain, stiffness and tenderness in joints, muscles, tendons and ligaments—but which does not inflame or damage tissues.

fibrositis: see *fibromyalgia*.

flare (or flare-up): an episode when arthritis symptoms return or worsen.

flexion contracture: the inability to fully extend a joint. This condition causes joints to stay bent; may be helped, or at least prevented from becoming worse, with stretching exercises.

genetic marker: the gene product, usually a protein, associated with a distinct trait. For instance, HLA-B27 is associated with a susceptibility to ankylosing spondylitis.

gold compounds: strong, slow-acting drugs used to treat rheumatoid arthritis, psoriatic arthritis and some cases of juvenile arthritis.

gout: a form of arthritis caused by deposits of uric acid crystals in the joints, usually in the feet and particularly the big toe; easily treated through medication and diet.

Heberden's nodes: bony growths that affect the joint nearest the fingernails; a symptom of osteoarthritis.

HLA: see *human leukocyte antigen.*

human leukocyte antigen: a system of genetic markers on the surfaces of cells that identify and fight specific invading organisms. Possessing or missing certain HLA genes has been found to be associated with particular types of arthritis.

hydrotherapy: using water to treat disorders—such as whirlpool massage for muscles or performing range of motion exercises in a pool.

immune system: a complex set of cells and proteins that defends the body against insults, such as a virus, infection, injury or transplanted organ.

infectious arthritis: a form of arthritis caused by infection of the joint by a bacterium, virus or fungus.

inflammation: body tissue's reaction to injury or disease; marked by swelling, redness, warmth and pain.

isometric exercise: an activity that strengthens a muscle by applying pressure against a stationary surface, without moving the involved joints—as when pressing the hands together.

isotonic exercise: strengthening moves that take a

joint through its full range of motion, as in calisthenics or weight training.

joint: the point where two or more bones meet.

joint capsule: the fibrous membrane that encloses the joint and bone ends.

juvenile arthritis: an umbrella term for all forms of arthritis when it occurs in children, who are affected differently than adults. Systemic juvenile rheumatoid arthritis is also known as Still's disease.

leukotrienes: chemicals released by white blood cells that cause inflammation.

ligament: strong bands of connective tissue that hold the bones of a joint together.

lupus: see *systemic lupus erythematosus.*

Lyme disease: a type of infectious arthritis, caused by the bite of a tick infected with an organism called *Borrelia burgdorferi.*

lymph nodes: small nodular glands that are part of the collection system for lymphatic fluid and lymphocytes.

lymphocyte: a type of white blood cell that has two forms: the B cell and T cell. The body increases production of lymphocytes when infection is present.

magnetic resonance imaging: also called MRI, a method of looking at different parts of the body to detect abnormalities. The equipment uses high-powered magnets rather than radiation to "photograph" areas.

nonsteroidal anti-inflammatory drugs (NSAIDs): medications that reduce inflammation by blocking prostaglandins, but do not contain corticosteroids. The category includes the nonprescription medication ibuprofen and prescription drugs such as fenoprofen, indomethacin, naproxen, phenylbutazone and tolmetin.

osteoarthritis: also called degenerative joint disease, the most common form of arthritis, in which joint cartilage breaks down.

osteotomy: surgically cutting or remodeling bone to improve joint alignment or weight distribution; an alternative to total joint replacement in selected patients.

pannus: in rheumatoid arthritis, overgrown synovium that invades the cartilage, and sometimes bone and ligaments.

penicillamine: one of the potent slow-acting drugs, prescribed for rheumatoid arthritis patients who do not respond well to other therapies.

polymyositis: muscle inflammation similar to dermatomyositis but without the skin rash.

prostaglandin: a hormone-like fatty acid found in the body that is involved in inflammation.

pseudogout: also called calcium pyrophosphate dihydrate crystal deposition, or CPPD, an arthritic condition caused by certain types of calcium crystals that enter and irritate joints, typically the knees.

psoriatic arthritis: a form of arthritis that occurs in association with psoriasis, a disorder that erupts in scaly red patches on the skin.

purines: compounds found in most proteins and also made in the body. A defect in the body's ability to handle purines is often the cause of gout.

RA: see *rheumatoid arthritis.*

range of motion: the full extent that a limb or other body part can be moved, in any direction or at any angle.

Raynaud's phenomenon: often the first symptom of scleroderma, a condition in which the blood supply to the extremities is reduced. Fingers or toes become "frostbitten"—pale and cold—in response to cool temperatures or emotional stress.

Reiter's syndrome: a form of arthritis linked to some bacterial infections and associated with the genetic marker HLA-B27. This condition affects the spine, and causes inflammations of the eye and urethra (the duct that drains urine from the bladder).

rheumatic disease: any of several disorders characterized by pain and inflammation in joints, connective tissue or muscles.

rheumatism: an older term used to refer to a variety of musculoskeletal problems.

rheumatoid arthritis: an autoimmune disease of unknown cause that brings pain, stiffness, inflammation and sometimes destruction of the joints, and may also affect lungs, skin, blood vessels and eyes.

scleroderma: a rheumatic disease involving abnormal deposits of collagen in the skin and other organs, which can cause them to thicken and harden.

sed rate: see *erythrocyte sedimentation rate.*

Sjögren's syndrome: a chronic autoimmune disorder that may accompany rheumatoid arthritis, lupus, scleroderma or other connective tissue diseases. The glands that produce tears and saliva become inflamed, causing dryness of the eyes and mouth.

SLE: see *systemic lupus erythematosus.*

slow-acting drugs: a group of powerful medications—such as antimalarials, gold compounds and penicillamine—that may take weeks or months to reduce or eliminate symptoms; prescribed in severe arthritis cases where anti-inflammatory drugs fail.

spondyloarthropathies: arthritic diseases that affect the spine, such as ankylosing spondylitis and Reiter's syndrome.

Still's disease: the systemic form of juvenile rheumatoid arthritis, which can affect the heart, lungs and blood. Symptoms include fever and skin rash as well as joint pain.

synovectomy: surgery to remove a synovium affected by inflammation.

synovial fluid: a clear, slippery fluid produced by the

synovium that lubricates joints and connective tissue so that they move smoothly and easily.

synovitis: inflammation of the synovium.

synovium: the membrane that lines the inside of freely moving joints.

systemic: affecting many systems of the body.

systemic lupus erythematosus (SLE): an autoimmune disorder that causes changes in connective tissue and can affect the skin, joints and internal organs.

T cell: a type of white blood cell that has been called the "conductor" of the immune system. These cells can prevent or help in the production of antibodies by B cells, or they can kill foreign invaders such as a virus or bacteria.

tendon: a fibrous, inelastic band of tissue that connects a muscle to bone.

tendonitis: inflammation of a tendon.

TENS: see *transcutaneous electrical nerve stimulator*.

thermotherapy: using heat as a pain-relief treatment, such as heating pads, hot water bottle or hot compresses.

tophi: lumps that form under the skin where urate crystals have deposited; a symptom of gout.

transcutaneous electrical nerve stimulator: a device placed on the skin that sends out a low electrical current. The tingling sensation relieves pain in joints or muscles.

urate crystal: the crystallized form of uric acid that collects in a joint, classically in the big toe, of people with gout, and triggers inflammation.

uric acid: a by-product of the breakdown of purines in proteins. The acid circulates in the bloodstream, then passes through the kidneys and is eliminated through the urine. Gout sufferers have high levels of uric acid in their blood.

vasculitis: a rheumatic disease with inflammation of the blood vessels.

Index